THE
WEIGH
TO WIN
AT WEIGHT
LOSS

THE
WEIGH TO WIN AT WEIGHT LOSS

LYNN HILL

FOUNDER OF WEIGH TO WIN, INC.

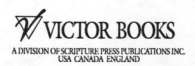

VICTOR BOOKS

A DIVISION OF SCRIPTURE PRESS PUBLICATIONS INC.
USA CANADA ENGLAND

All Scripture references are from the *Holy Bible, New International Version,* © 1973, 1978, 1984, International Bible Society. Used by permission of Zondervan Bible Publishers.

Copyediting: Carole S. Streeter
Cover Design: Scott Rattray
Back Cover Photo: Gary Mester

Library of Congress Cataloging-in-Publication Data

Hill, Lynn 1950 –
    The Weigh to Win at weight loss / by Lynn Hill.
      p.   cm.
    Includes bibliographical references.
    ISBN 0-89693-059-9
    1. Reducing. 2. Christian life. 3. Obesity –
Religious aspects – Christianity. I. Weigh to Win,
Inc. II. Title
  RM222.2.H473 1992
  613.2'5 – dc20   92-3730
                                           CIP

3 4 5 6 7 8 9 10 Printing/Year 96 95 94 93 92

*To my family
with love and a thankful heart*

Contents

Foreword

Going on a diet is not the answer to losing weight.

"What? I thought that dieting was the only way a person could lose weight."

The problem with this thinking is that if you have to go "on" a diet, you will probably have to go "off" of it eventually, and you will regain the weight you previously lost.

Lynn Hill is living proof that going "on" diets such as liquid diet drinks, starvation diets, grapefruit diets, and other fad diets, or resorting to diet aids such as pills, fiber supplements, appetite suppressing candies, and expensive prepackaged diet foods, does not work in the long run.

"So, if going on a diet is not the answer, what is?"

The *Weigh to Win Weight Management System* and the program contained in this book provide a fresh, positive Christian perspective to weight loss. This comes as no surprise, since Lynn's desire is to reach out to discouraged, hopeless, or guilt-ridden individuals who struggle with being overweight and who are looking for solutions.

The Weigh to Win at Weight Loss reveals the reasons behind overeating, as well as exposing the poor eating behaviors which have resulted. Lynn offers many very practical principles for overcoming poor behaviors and replacing them with healthy ones. Lynn's personal experience and encouraging insights are what bring the book to life.

This book expresses Lynn's passion—to help others succeed at losing weight and keeping it off! Lynn points the way to a road of freedom—freedom from diets, freedom from guilt, and freedom in Christ to live a healthier lifestyle. Her heart's desire is to pass on some of the encouragement that God has given to her while traveling down the road to freedom.

Whether you are 10 pounds, 50 pounds, or 250 pounds overweight, dealing with people who struggle with being overweight, or just interested in learning a healthier lifestyle, Lynn's book and her *Weigh to Win Weight Management System* can draw you away from the diet mentality and get you started down your own road to freedom.

MARLA SMITH
Registered Dietitian

INTRODUCTION

My Personal Weight-Loss Journey

Did you know that all diets work and all weight loss programs work? You have probably been able to lose at least some weight on every diet you have tried. But, to lose weight *and* to maintain that weight loss, you have to find a food plan and a life plan which has variety and flexibility, is not boring, and is suited to your unique needs on a daily basis.

During my twenty years of being overweight, I tried every diet that "came down the pike." I knew the basics of nutrition. I could quote the basic food groups and knew what I should and should not eat. So just being informed about nutrition was not the answer.

☐ I told myself that food, in general, was my problem. Therefore, to overcome the problem I would have to give up food. I tried starvation, praying to the Lord to help me be strong and gain victory over my need for food. However, along with any weight I lost, I was also losing the joy of living. I became irritable with my family. I was angry with my fat body. I hated being hungry all the time. When the hunger was no longer bearable, I would binge on anything and everything available, while berating myself for being hopelessly fat and ugly, for being undisciplined, and for being out of control.

☐ Next, I thought I could handle the hunger if I just took some of those pills which were available at every grocery store, drug store, and variety store. I would just pick up a package to "get me over the hump." But I found that I could eat even with my body full of appetite suppressants! What I did not realize then was that I was not eating because I was hungry; I was eating as an emotional response to life events, a learned response which had become an ingrained habit. The diet pills made me nervous and made my heart beat rapidly. I was just as irritable as ever, and tears came easily as I once again felt there was no hope.

I have always been an organizer. Almost every area of my life was controlled and scheduled; my weight was the one part of my life which refused discipline and control, and I could not figure out why. Yet, I was sure that I could devise a manageable plan if I just worked a little harder.

☐ Eventually, I decided that starvation with or without pills was not the answer. All I needed was a little food to keep me from getting hungry. The liquid protein drink fad was in full swing with a whole array of shake mixes which could be fixed in a variety of ways. Each promised that after just a little while, I would not be hungry, and yet the 400 calories per day diet would make the fat rapidly fall off. In no time at all I would look thin and beautiful. How I looked was not as important to me as how I felt. I felt like a failure. For four months I ate no food and faithfully drank my drink. I was so strong. At church potlucks I would busy myself with the cleanup so people would not notice I was not eating. I thanked the Lord for "helping me to be strong." What I did not realize was that God does not honor foolishness. When I became thoroughly bored with the diet drink and fed up with the lack of variety, I went off the diet, not having learned anything about the control of food—something I so longed to achieve. The forty pounds I had lost were back on in a matter of weeks, plus more.

☐ "The Lord was helping me to be so strong! Why did He give up on me?" I questioned. Still determined to find an answer, several of us in our church formed a Bible study to deal with our problem of overeating. We found some materials in our local Christian bookstore and delved in earnestly. Surely this would be the answer. The materials told me that I had to repent of "fleshly indulgence" in the name of Jesus Christ and that He would not allow me to fail. The study told me that lust for food would never be satisfied and that "unbridled lust" for food was as sinful as unbridled lust for someone's body.

I would pray, ask for forgiveness, tell the Lord I wanted Him to have control of my life and my eating, and then as soon as I got home I would sit down with a whole package of potato chips and a pint of dip. I felt that I must be a terrible sinner and that God could not possibly love me. The materials said God would not let me fail, and yet here I was—stuffing my face.

My husband was pastor of the church. I was up to my ears in church activities. I loved the Lord Jesus Christ and had accepted Him as my personal Savior. I tried my best to be a good Christian example, but the size of my body seemed to overshadow any evidence of Christ in my life and contradict my Christian testimony. I felt like a substandard Christian. Each week's Bible study left me feeling more spiritually defeated.

I read many other books about weight loss from a Christian point of view. All of them seemed to come to the same conclusion—if you are overweight, you are sinning because you are allowing food to take the place God should rightfully have in your life. "God, You are Lord of my life!" I cried out in agony. "But I eat food without even realizing I am eating. I look down and find an empty wrapper and realize I have just eaten a dozen cookies. What am I to do?"

☐ I joined a local weight loss support group because I began to realize that I could not do this on my own. I thought paying a weekly fee would help to motivate me. It did. However, the food plan was complicated, and alcoholic drinks were used in many recipes. I knew that alcohol was high in calories and of virtually no nutritional value. The use of alcohol can weaken one's resolve to make healthy food choices. Since there are so many problems associated with the abuse of alcohol, I did not feel its use was appropriate in a food plan which was supposed to encourage healthy eating. The program said I could have potato chips, but who stops at ten potato chips? Not me! If the bag is open, it will be empty. I dropped out, gained weight, joined again, and dropped out again.

☐ In desperation, I decided that I just had not been paying enough to lose weight. Still considering food my problem, I enrolled in one of those expensive programs where you buy special prepackaged foods. Although we were on a limited pastoral income, my husband supported me in the decision. He could see my pain and just wanted me to be happy. My prepackaged foods cost more than it did to feed the other three members of my family. I was willing to make the financial sacrifice, no matter what, and felt "the Lord would provide a way" because I was doing this to achieve discipline over my sinful eating. I *was* losing weight, but after several months, the monotony of the food choices available, the difficulty of having to prepare separate meals for myself, and the financial hardship became just too great. Once again, nothing had really changed. I had learned well how to eat those special foods, but I had not learned how to live with real food in the real world. I again regained all the weight I had lost, plus more.

☐ Off and on through the years I would give up on losing weight. I would become indifferent and decide that people would just have to like me the way I was. The problem was that I did not like myself the way I was. I hated shopping for size 24¹/₂ dresses. I hated wearing clothes that hurt. I hated not being able to take my children to an amusement park because I might not be able to make it through the turnstiles. The thought that I must be a sinner continued to nag at me, keeping my self-esteem low and my spirit crushed.

Then I slipped into a severe depression, precipitated largely by the long, dark winters in Fairbanks, Alaska, where my husband was an associate pastor. Unless one has experienced them, one cannot truly understand how dark the Alaskan winters are and how long they last. I was malnourished from fad dieting, and overtired from trying to meet deadlines for opening a child-care center for our church; also, I later discovered that my body is chemically sensitive to extremes of darkness. With the return of light, rest, and eating instead of starving, I was able to overcome the depression. My husband and I knew that as much as we loved the people and scenery of Alaska, I would not be able to tolerate another winter. We packed up what we could get in the back of a pickup truck and took off with our two children on the 4,000-mile journey to my hometown of Plymouth, Indiana.

□ After nearly a year of getting settled in, I started feeling the need to do something about my weight which had climbed to over 250 pounds. I began the old inner debate with, "Nothing has ever worked before, and it is not going to work now. So why should I put myself through it again just to fail? No matter how hard I have tried, the weight keeps coming back. And as long as I am overweight, I am failing God and my family. God cannot possibly love me fat. It is hopeless."

Then, for a moment, I became silent. For a moment, I stopped pleading with the Lord to remove my desire to overeat, stopped begging Him to take all the tempting foods away, stopped bombarding heaven with my promises to lose weight. Then He came in a still, small voice and said, "Lynn, I look at your heart." He let me know He loved me *fat!* What about all the books that emphasized the sin of gluttony? What about conquering my "fleshly indulgence"? What about my "lust for food"? And then it came to me, that the only one giving me those negative messages was the devil, who wanted to keep me in bondage to low self-esteem and a crushed spirit. Oh, what a deceiver Satan is!

At that moment, the Lord began a process in me which confirmed, once and for all, that *I did not eat out of fleshly indulgence or lust for food. I had learned to overeat.* Systematically and culturally I had been taught to overeat. Those learned behaviors had been subtly wrapping around me like a cobweb which had turned into a cable. What I had learned was so ingrained that it would take years, even a lifetime, to overcome.

God let me know that *I would have to take the first step.* I would have to show Him that I did not want to just be thin but also to be healthy; that I was willing to work on changing those learned habits, not just for a while, but for a lifetime.

A quiet realization and determination took over, and yet mixed in was true fear. I was terrified of failure. How could it be any different this time?

For one thing, I had had enough experience with many of the weight loss programs on the market to know what would work and what would not. God carefully revealed to me that He had provided a whole variety of fruits, vegetables, meats, and grains on this earth and that He had not created them for me to avoid. Those foods had a purpose for my body, but I had to learn to use them wisely. I asked Him to guide me in my food choices, acknowledging that He was not going to take a hot fudge sundae out of my hands if I chose to eat it. I had to tell Him, "Lord, *I* am going to resist this hot fudge sundae with *Your* help." He has never failed to provide His help for me.

I love to cook. Therefore I needed to find some plan which would allow me to cook when I wanted to, but which was also easy to follow if I came home tired and just wanted to grab something quick to eat from the refrigerator.

My work schedule required frequent meals at restaurants. How could I follow a specific food plan and still eat out?

I did not want to count calories the rest of my life. Pills, meal replacements, and supplements had obviously never worked. So, where was I to begin to find a program which *would* work?

I joined a local support group because I felt the need to have others around me who understood the struggle I was facing. I also humbly acknowledged the need to face those scales each week. Being accountable to someone else, a group, a family member, or a good friend is very often critical to successful weight loss. If I could have done it on my own, I would not have been struggling all these years. My hands were shaking as I filled out the registration papers required by the group. I stood in the weigh-in line with dread and yet felt the Lord was there with me. I prayed a prayer and told the Lord that I was afraid that I might fail again. I acknowledged I had to do the work, and promised that if He would be there to give me strength, I would give Him the credit for *our* success.

☐ I began my research for the "perfect" program. No *"Lose Ten Pounds in Ten Days"* diets for me this time. I wanted facts. The Food and Drug Administration, American Dietetic Association, American Diabetic Association, the *Journal of American Medicine,* and other well-documented and well-researched studies helped me to put together the Rainbow Food Plan. *No calorie counting,* because I knew I would not do it for a lifetime. *No more pills or diet shakes.* I wanted something safe. *No more cooking separate meals.* If it was healthy for me, it had to be healthy, as well as palatable, for my family too. It had to be easy to do whether at home, at Mom's, or at a restaurant.

I followed this food plan faithfully. Sure, I made mistakes sometimes and went back to some old eating habits, but I did not allow these mistakes to make me go "off" of my Rainbow Food Plan. Mistakes were merely costly detours. I had a high level of energy. There were many foods I could eat, so I did not go hungry. The Rainbow Food Plan worked for me and I lost 120 pounds in one year!

☐ When I reached my goal weight on March 16, 1987, the Lord reminded me of my promise to give Him the credit for our success. He said, "Lynn, this program has worked for you and it can work for other people too." I started a *Weigh to Win* class with six people in my home on June

1, 1987. Within a few weeks the group had outgrown my home and began meeting in local churches. I soon gave up my full-time job and started teaching seven *Weigh to Win* classes a week.

For the next three years, I trained instructors who worked to open classes in several states. Thousands of people were being helped by the Rainbow Food Plan the Lord had led me to develop. With a dedicated staff and an advisory board of directors, *Weigh to Win* has continued to grow steadily over the years.

In November 1990, through an article which I wrote for *Guideposts* magazine, I received thousands of phone calls and letters. People told me of their pain and their feelings of worthlessness. They told how they felt God could not possibly love them. I knew and understood. How could I reach these people with the *Weigh to Win* message? We could not train instructors fast enough to meet the crying need.

Two years ago, I felt the Lord nudging me to provide a way for individuals to participate in the *Weigh to Win* program on their own or by forming support groups. Ideas poured into my mind on how to accomplish this task while maintaining the top quality program *Weigh to Win* had become. I realized that implementing these ideas would require nationwide exposure, which we did not have at the time. So I pushed the ideas aside until the Lord revealed what He would have me to do. The *Guideposts* article gave *Weigh to Win* the exposure we needed and soon people were crying for our help. I took those ideas which had been mentally pushed aside two years ago and put them into action to develop the *Weigh to Win Weight Management System*. The system's materials are designed to give people everything they need to be successful with their weight loss once and for all, with or without the help of a trained *Weigh to Win* instructor.

Professionally recorded cassette tapes allow me to teach hundreds of support groups across the country. I can also go along with individuals via cassette tape as they get in their cars or work around the house, to motivate and share what I have learned through these years. What a joy to hear from people all over the country who are "Weigh to Winners."

Now the outcry has been heard for a book that tells how I lost weight, but also gives a "how to" for all of you who struggle with a weight problem. You need information, education, a road map to follow, and motivation to accomplish your goal. Years of research and study have gone into this book. So have a lot of love and caring. Even if you have failed at every weight-loss diet you have ever tried, remember that you only really fail when you give up trying. *Weigh to Win* will give you the hope you need and a way to *win* at weight loss once and for all!

LYNN HILL
Plymouth, Indiana

ONE

The Psychology of Overeating

We are our bodies. We are not split into physical and psychological organisms. It would be easier if we could separate our physical needs from our emotional ones, but we come as a package deal, and often the two are intermingled.

Most of us have believed that willpower is the cure for overeating, and we hate ourselves when we weaken. Yes, it does take an act of will to make a choice between sugar-free gelatin or a piece of peanut butter cream pie, but sometimes our learned behaviors interfere with our willpower.

Our Use of Food Is Learned Behavior

We have learned to use food as our comforter and stress reliever. Without being aware of it, we develop a relationship with food that makes it difficult for us to handle stress, depression, anger, or loneliness without turning to food. We have not learned to defer gratification or turn to other means to meet those emotional needs.

How do we learn to use food to deal with our emotional needs? How do we use food without even being aware of its place in our lives? Let us start with this scenario:

An eighteen-month-old child begins sobbing and crying. The parent is talking with a friend on the phone and needs for the child to stop crying so the conversation can resume.

The parent hurriedly places a bottle of juice in her mouth. With tears still flowing, she accepts the food in place of having her needs met.

The child may have been physically hungry and the bottle did satisfy a legitimate need. However, what if she had just pinched a finger? The bottle teaches that *food is the response to pain*. What if her four-year-old sibling had just taken away a favorite toy? The bottle teaches that *food is the response to loss*. What if she had just realized that the parent had left to go answer the phone and she was left alone? The bottle teaches that *food is the response to loneliness*. What if her diaper had just been soiled? The bottle teaches that *food is the response to discomfort*. What if she just needed to be hugged and cuddled? The bottle teaches that *food is love*.

As the child grows, other situations reinforce the use of food in response to emotions. She goes to the doctor for an immunization shot and is given a sucker. She falls off a bike, skins a knee, goes home, is given a cookie and told, "Here, this will make it better—stop crying." *Food is the response to pain*.

Other factors begin to form learned behaviors. The child is told, "Eat everything on your plate." So she learns to eat, even though there is no physical hunger. "If you eat your spinach, you may have dessert." So she learns that *food is the response or reward for tolerating something she does not like*. When the child is active and restless, the baby-sitter places a plate of cookies and a glass of milk on the table, saying, "Here, this will keep you busy for a while." She learns that *food is the response to boredom*.

Because my father was very ambitious and received numerous promotions requiring our family to relocate every year or two, I attended fourteen different schools during my childhood. I remember often feeling lonely and apprehensive about attending yet another school and trying to make new friends. I am sure my mother had her share of apprehensions about getting settled in a new house, trying to find a church home, and budgeting for the expenses of a move. Mom and I would head for the kitchen and bake away our loneliness and fears. At least for a little while, we could shut out the new faces and places which would soon become part of our lives.

Soup commercials on television say to give a "mug and a hug," further associating food with love. Just after you have finished a meal, you stop by the home of a close friend and she says, "But I fixed this pecan pie just for you, because I know it is your favorite." If you refuse the pie, you're afraid your friend will think you don't appreciate her effort to show you how much you are loved.

Food is frequently associated with the good things in life. What is a ball game without a hot dog or a party without pizza? What is a birthday without cake and ice cream, or Thanksgiving without pumpkin pie à la mode? What is a church without potluck dinners? What is a Sunday School class without Kool-Aid and cookies for the children and donuts and coffee for the adults?

Food is a reward for good behavior. The parent says to the child, "Sit still in church and I will give you a piece of candy when we get in the car." Or, "With that great report card you deserve an ice cream cone."

My son is a top-notch Bible quizzer, and many times at the meets I hear coaches bribe the teens with, "Just get one question this round, and I will buy you a candy bar," or "Win this round and I will take you out for all the pizza you can chow down." Why not say, "Win this round and we will go bowling, or roller skating, or sledding, or have a bike race, or an overnight at the coach's house"?

Food Becomes the Answer for All of Our Emotions

If food is the answer to feeling sad, lonely, depressed, stressful, bored, or hurting, and if food is also the answer for all the good times in our lives, then food must be the answer for *all* of our emotions. *Food is for when we feel bad, and food is for when we feel good.* Most of us are either feeling bad or good all the time. I do not think anyone gets up in the morning and says, "I feel indifferent today." So we go through life unconsciously using food as a learned response to normal life events.

Like the child enduring his spinach, after completing each of my most dreaded household chores, I used to reward myself with something from the refrigerator. I would vacuum and then eat some cookies. I would clean the bathroom and that was worth a whole dish of ice cream. And so on, until I had eaten my way through the housework.

When my husband had to be away, I was drawn to the kitchen. When the children started "getting on my nerves," I would eat. When the bills piled up and there was not enough money to go around, food let me put the pressure out of my mind for a while. I could even eat when I was sick.

Using Food Inappropriately Is Not a Spiritual Problem

"But I thought God was the answer for all of life's ups and downs." I agree, He is. However, by adulthood our learned behaviors are so ingrained in us that our use of food is a habit. We have learned to pray and rely on God to meet our needs, and we want Him to have first place in our lives. But we have also learned to use food to handle our emotional needs. Using food inappropriately to delay dealing with our feelings is not a spiritual problem; rather, it is learned behavior so ingrained in us that it can be overcome only through awareness, education, and the Lord's help and direction.

Revelation 2:17 says, "To him who overcomes, I will give some of the hidden manna." If we will work hard to overcome these habits, we may receive some of God's "hidden manna." I can just imagine how wonderful eating food from His table must be. I doubt that the manna from God's table would be loaded with fat and calories. When we have overcome the learned habits that make us want those high fat and high calorie foods, then we will be ready for the healthy manna, physically and spiritually, which the Lord is ready and waiting to give us.

Two
Facing Reality

The first step in overcoming a problem is recognizing that we have one. I have heard it said that overweight people see themselves from the neck up. I suppose that is true at times. I saw my fat body in store windows, but I would instantly look away, denying the reflection in the window.

I went through countless times of denial when I decided that I was "born to be fat," and everyone would just have to like it or lump it. Much of my feeling of denial stemmed from the fact that I did not know how to be anything but fat. Every time I had tried to lose weight I had failed.

Denial

You are in a stage of denial when you make comments like:

☐ "I will start dieting tomorrow." (Tomorrow never comes.)

☐ "All I need is willpower."

☐ "I really do not eat much at all. I don't know why I gain weight."

☐ "I cannot lose weight with a skinny spouse who can eat everything and not gain an ounce."

☐ "I cannot afford the 'right' foods to lose weight."

☐ "You would be overweight too, if you had the problems I have."

One *Weigh to Win* member who was struggling with her weight shared with the group that she had a terrible problem resisting peach cobbler. In fact, she had eaten several portions over the last few weeks. The support group leader asked to look at her Weekly Food Record to see if she could determine exactly what the class member was eating. The leader noted that no peach cobbler was listed anywhere on the sheet. The member responded with, "Oh, I don't write down the things I am not supposed to eat." That is a sure sign of denial!

A woman at church jarred me into reality one Sunday when we were discussing how navy and black colors made us look thinner. She said her mother used to tell her, "Even a barn painted black is still a barn." That statement did something to me. I thought, "If I am going to be a barn, I am going to be a bright one." I went out and bought a hot pink sweater with purple slacks and a sunny yellow sweater with light beige slacks. Those colors so improved my outlook and how I felt about myself that they helped to trigger my successful weight loss which began about three months later.

Making Bargains

When moments of reality seep into your consciousness, you begin to make bargains with yourself, with your family, and with God.

☐ "I will just cut back on my portions."

☐ "I will diet on Monday through Thursday and then eat anything I want on the weekends."

☐ "I will join a health spa. All I really need is exercise."

☐ "When things slow down at work, I will get started."

☐ "I will buy an exercise bike."

☐ "I will take diet pills."

☐ "I will have my stomach stapled."

☐ "I will spend $3,000 and drink liquid drinks for weeks."

☐ "God, You take away my desire to overeat, and we will have this problem licked in no time."

You may become depressed and angry because you have "let yourself go," angry that others seem to be able to eat anything they want and still lose weight, upset about the dates you did not have in high school. You may become depressed about how long it is going to take to lose weight, or about how hard you think it is going to be to lose weight; depressed because you think you are going to have to eat foods you hate in order to lose weight; and depressed about the realization that your future health and the quality of life you hope for may be at stake.

Although I am not a trained psychologist, I recognize the psychological implications of the questions which follow. I find my own thoughts and actions revealed in some of them. Many of the people I love and care for are still struggling with others. Take just a moment to complete this Self-Evaluation Questionnaire. Make this a time of measuring where you are right now, but do not be too hard on yourself. Remember that overcoming the habits which have caused you to overeat is a process. There are no right or wrong answers to these questions.

SELF-EVALUATION QUESTIONNAIRE

	Yes	No
1. Do you feel guilty about eating?	___	___
2. Do you eat large amounts of junk food?	___	___
3. Do you hide food? Or hide from others while eating?	___	___
4. Do you eat to the point of nausea and vomiting?	___	___
5. Would you rather be cooking than doing almost anything else?	___	___
6. Have you forced vomiting?	___	___
7. Do you take laxatives to control weight?	___	___
8. Do you weigh on a scale more than once a week?	___	___
9. Have you found yourself unable to stop eating?	___	___
10. Do you use starvation to control weight?	___	___
11. Do you consider the way you have been eating normal?	___	___
12. Do you eat until your stomach hurts?	___	___
13. Do certain occasions call for certain foods? (like movies and popcorn)	___	___
14. In your lifetime, have you lost more than fifty pounds?	___	___
15. Does a "good" restaurant serve large portions?	___	___

	Yes	No
16. Do you eat snacks before going out to eat with others?	——	——
17. Do you eat faster than other people?	——	——
18. Do you wake up at night to eat?	——	——

Do not let your responses to these questions get you down; I can promise you that there is hope for you. Had I taken this test before I lost my excess weight, my answers to many of the questions would have been yes. Now, with God's help, I can truthfully say NO, NO, NO to all the questions except the one about having lost fifty pounds in my lifetime, and this is now a resounding, happy YES!

One Step at a Time

Look at the places you answered yes and take steps to work on them one at a time. Do not be unrealistic and think you are going to change everything overnight. Pick out one area which is a problem for you and spend a week or a month working on it—however long it takes to overcome the problem. You may find yourself standing in front of the refrigerator, secretively nibbling on something, when you suddenly become aware of what you are doing. Thank the Lord for bringing the problem to your attention, and then *get out of the kitchen!* If you find yourself eating until your stomach hurts, make a conscious effort to slow your eating and stop when you feel satisfied without feeling "stuffed."

Many of your responses can probably be traced to your emotions. The behaviors which cause you to turn to food in response to emotions are learned. Overcoming these learned responses is a step-by-step process. Sometimes you will do well, and other times you will revert back to your old behavior, because the path of overeating is more familiar and more comfortable than this new path of healthy eating.

If your eating is or has been out of control, it is important to realize that God wants the very best for you and this means a healthy body. Illness and other health problems are not in His plan.

Learning new responses to old habits is a process. God cannot do the changing for you—you must take *action*. He also does not condemn you when you make mistakes, but He does want you to *keep on trying*.

> "For I know the plans I have for you," declares the Lord, "plans to prosper you and not to harm you, plans to give you hope and a future. Then you will call upon Me and come and pray to Me, and I will listen to you. You will seek Me and find Me when you seek Me with all your heart. I will be found by you," declares the Lord, "and will bring you back from captivity" (Jeremiah 29:11-14).

Are you being held in captivity by food? God will not take a bag of cookies out of your hands but, if you will listen to His small, quiet voice, He will teach you a better way and "bring you back from captivity." God bless you, dear one. I care about *you!*

A Special Note

If you struggle with the use of pills, laxatives, and vomiting to control your weight, I urge you to seek the help of a Christian counselor and physician to overcome this problem. The *Weigh to Win Weight Management System* can help you with making healthy food choices, but the use of pills, laxatives, and vomiting will only sabotage your success and endanger your health. I plead with you to take action and get professional help now. Let us work together to make you a whole, healthy person—physically, emotionally, and spiritually.

Three

Is Overeating a Sin?

The following is typical of the many letters which I receive daily:

Dear Mrs. Hill,

I went to the doctor last Monday. I weighed in at 241 pounds, the most I have ever weighed. I have been overweight all of my life. My parents are overweight. My mother's greatest joy is for someone to eat and enjoy her cooking. I have two older sisters, both overweight.

I have been on liquid protein diets, Dr. Dumbo's low-carbohydrate diet (eat all meats — I was in heaven — but I didn't lose weight), Weight Watcher's, and Overeaters Victorious. I have tried diet pills, Slimfast, and starving. I've lost at least one whole person and gained it back and more. I thought Overeaters Victorious was my answer because it was based on the Bible and was a Christian support group. The group dwindled down until there were only two of us. The rest gave up. Finally we did too. I was worse off than I was before because most of the Scriptures dealt with the sin of gluttony and our appetite being our god. I have been so guilt-ridden since then that all I do is eat. I have a fear that I am going to be left behind when Jesus raptures the church because I am so disobedient in this area. I beg for forgiveness daily because my eating is out of control. I *hate myself* and wonder how can Jesus possibly love me when I repeatedly willfully sin.

My doctor told me that if I continued on the trend of gaining, I would be over 300 pounds by the time I am forty. I cried and cried, prayed and prayed. I made up my mind for the thousandth time that I was going to do something about my weight. I did all right last week, but since the weekend I've blown it. I tried to fast Monday (to punish myself for bingeing), but I couldn't make it through lunch. I've cried a river—my back and legs hurt—I look repulsive. Thank God my husband is very loving and kind to me. He tries to help, and never criticizes when I fail.

When my *Guideposts* came yesterday (after I blew my fast), I thought, "Maybe there is something in there to help me"—I don't know why I thought that. I didn't get to your article until today. I felt like maybe God put that thought in my mind so I would write you. Whether or not I ever lose weight, I need to know that God loves me. . . . I can't deal with this overwhelming guilt any longer. Maybe if I didn't feel that my salvation and forgiveness of sins was dependent on my weight or weight loss, I could deal with the problem without so much fear of failure. Right now I am afraid that if I don't lose weight, not only will I be fat and ugly the rest of my life, but I am afraid I will lose my salvation because I am a willful disobedient sinner. Please help me if you can.

Dear one, I have good news for you! The one making you feel guilty is the deceiver Satan. First Samuel 16:7 says, "The

Lord does not look at the things man looks at. Man looks at the outward appearance, but the Lord looks at the heart." All you need to know is that your heart belongs to the Lord. Let go of your guilt!

Yes, your eating is out of control. Yes, you turn to food as a response to life events and emotional turmoil. But you have *learned* to use food in this way. It has become a habit. It does not mean that you are willfully disobedient. Habits are very hard to break—especially when we have been taught from birth to use food for something it is not. How many times have you found yourself eating and you did not even realize you were? How can it be a willful disobedience when the habit was so strong that you reacted without conscious awareness? God loves you just as you are. John 3:16 says, "For God so loved the world [you] that He gave His one and only Son, that *whoever* [He doesn't make overweight persons an exception] believes in Him shall not perish but have eternal life." All you have to do is ask that your sins be forgiven and believe in the Lord. God has promised that He does not look at our outward appearance.

What about the Sin of Gluttony?

As for the sin of gluttony, do you realize how little mention of the word *glutton* or *gluttony* is in the Bible? *Strong's Exhaustive Concordance* only lists four references and those are mostly concerning the behavior of pagans who were also involved in orgies, drunkenness, and sexual immorality—you know, "fleshly indulgence." The gluttons of biblical times were people who would have huge feasts and banquets at which they would stuff themselves with food and then go and vomit just to be able to stuff themselves again. I would say that their stuffing themselves for pure fleshly pleasure was a sin. However, I do not know any overweight persons who stuff themselves out of pure fleshly pleasure. We eat as a learned response, not just for the pure pleasure of eating. Even those who are bulimic may stuff themselves and then go and vomit, but they do not do it so they can go and immediately stuff themselves again. Persons suffering from bulimia will vomit or purge out of the guilt they feel for having eaten. The amount of food eaten may not even be very much.

Yes, Philippians 4:3 says, "Their god is their stomach," but this passage is talking about the enemies of the cross of Christ. Dear Christian friend, you are not an enemy of the cross—you are an ally. You know God is the Lord of your life. You have some habits which the Lord would like for you to get under control, but your stomach is not your god.

Has it done you any good to think about your overeating as a sin? Has it really helped you gain control over the problem? Or has it left you defeated spiritually? Would God want you to be defeated over body fat? No, but Satan would like for that to happen.

Well-intentioned Christians have published much information on weight loss from points of view quite opposite to the one I am presenting in this book. I challenge you to ask yourself what such viewpoints accomplish. God asks us to come to Him just as we are. The familiar song, "Just As I Am" says everything about God's love and acceptance, whether we are built like a Saint Bernard or a Chihuahua.

Weakness Is Not Necessarily Wickedness

I believe the human body is a temple of God; with that realization there comes a responsibility to take care of it. But our salvation does not depend on our ability to overcome a lifelong food habit. Overeating is not a hell-sending sin. Weakness is not necessarily wickedness. Yes, we need to keep working on gaining control of our eating but, if we make a mistake and temporarily slip back into an old eating habit because it is familiar and comfortable to us, it will not cost us our salvation. We just need to get right back to doing what we must do to conquer the problem. We fail only when we give up trying.

I remember feeling just like the writer of the letter. I remember the guilt and despair. I remember the fear of failure and the disgust with myself. I remember thinking God could not possibly love me. I remember hating myself for eating a cookie. I remember thinking I had to punish my body into submission through starvation and pills. I remember going through the motions of being a pastor's wife, all the time feeling that I was failing as a Christian.

When I let the Lord really speak to me, the message I heard set me free. "I look at the heart," He said, and my spirit soared. I no longer needed to be chained down with guilt. God loved me—fat and all. Then, free of guilt, I wanted to be everything He would have me to be. Taking care of my body was part of that, not by starving or drinking diet drinks or taking pills—God does not honor foolishness—but by taking advantage of the wonderful variety of foods He has provided.

Jesus said, "The thief comes only to steal and kill and destroy; I have come that they may have life, and have it to the full" (John 10:10). Do not let Satan, the thief, steal your joy and destroy your spirit. Jesus wants you to have life and "have it to the full!"

Four

The "Now" Fixation

I am definitely a "now" person. When my brother went through a bone marrow transplant for cancer, I wanted him to be well "now." The treatment took many months. When we bought a century-old, dilapidated Victorian home, I wanted to make it into our dream house "now." So far it has been eight years, and we still have plenty of work to do. I have a bad back and am not supposed to lift anything heavy. However, when I get in the mood to rearrange the furniture I cannot seem to wait for my husband to get home, and the "now" fixation causes me to pay the price. I want my church to grow "now." I want the world to be at peace "now."

Most of us who have a weight problem suffer from the "now's." We want everything "now." If it takes longer than four days to lose our weight, we give up. You have probably heard the expression, "Lord, give me patience and do it *now*."

Unrealistic Goal-Setting

This "now" fixation usually teams up with another attitude which get us into trouble: unrealistic goal-setting which leads to self-criticism.

So many times I had said, "I am going to lose this weight, even if I have to starve." Of course, I could not go hungry very long, and soon I was back to overeating and gaining back any weight I had managed to lose—plus more, because I felt so guilty about failing. I did not want to accept the fact that healthy weight loss involved a steady, day-by-day commitment to a balanced diet. I wanted the fat off *now*.

To be successful, I had to realistically look at what had to be accomplished. Giving up on the idea of a "quick and easy" weight loss was not easy. However, concentrating on losing weight through hard work, planning, and a sensible weight loss program became the commitment I needed to succeed. The development of the *Weigh to Win Weight Management System* helped me to face the facts about long-term weight loss and maintenance of that weight loss.

To lose a pound of fat you must burn about 3,500 calories more than you eat. I am angered by the claims of some weight loss clinics which promise weight losses of five or more pounds per week. It is absurd to think that an average 160-pound person who may need 2,300 calories a day could possibly lose a pound of fat a day for weeks at a time.

If you weighed 160 pounds and ate a meager 800 calories per day, your calorie deficit would run about 1,500 calories each day, equal to three pounds of weight loss per week. Many of these programs promise excessive amounts of weight loss, but fail to mention that part of each pound lost is water and muscle loss—not just fat being burned. And then, when you fail to lose five pounds per week, they try to sell you pills and supplements which supposedly make your body burn fat more quickly. It is true that initially there may be a rapid loss of water weight for many people, sometimes as much as fifteen pounds in the first few days. After that, the weight comes off slowly, sometimes with temporary retention of fluid and an apparent weight gain.

If you follow the *Weigh to Win Weight Management System,* you will lose fat every day. Be honest with yourself. If you know for certain that you are being faithful to the Rainbow Food Plan, the stubborn weight may be nothing but water and salt retention or a metabolic change which occurs in some individuals—especially those who have been on very low calorie diets in the past. Either condition usually responds to extra water intake, a decrease in salt or high sodium foods, and an increase in activity levels.

The water gain phenomenon is one which has caused many "now" dieters to go off their weight loss program because of discouragement. One *Weigh to Win* member showed a three-pound gain at the scale. He was devastated. In looking at his diary sheet, I found he had eaten popcorn every night during the week. He also had salted the popcorn. When he quit salting the popcorn, he saw a good weight loss over the next couple of weeks.

Setting unrealistic goals is a sure way to set yourself up for failure. Be happy with an average weight loss of one-half to two pounds per week. It is encouraging to count down about six weeks on your calendar and set a goal of how many pounds you would like to lose in that amount of time. When I have done this in support groups, I can almost always predict the people who are going to be successful because they set a realistic goal of three or four pounds for the six weeks. Those who struggle with the "now's" set goals of ten to twenty pounds. It is better to set a smaller goal and meet or exceed it than to set a goal which would be difficult to meet.

Through my weight loss, I could not look at the whole picture of having to lose 120 pounds. I could handle it better by taking my weight loss in ten-pound increments. Each time I passed another ten-pound goal, I felt satisfaction that I was making progress.

Admitting Your Mistakes

Be honest with yourself and admit it when you make a mistake. If you have made a bad choice or a few bad choices during the week, admit it and then look at it as an opportunity to evaluate how things could be handled differently next week.

Write down on your Weekly Food Record what you ate — ignoring it will not make the extra calories go away. Having to write it down will make you think twice before making the same bad choice a second time.

Be honest with your support group leader, family, and friends. They are for you, not against you, and will understand that we all make mistakes sometimes. If you have made a mistake, discuss how you can work together to overcome your weight problem.

When you make a mistake, you should acknowledge that you are only human and then learn from the mistake. Do not let one little detour destroy all the good feelings you have had about the pounds you have already lost. Do not let other people make you feel guilty, either. Be assertive. Admit you made a mistake and take responsibility for it.

Setting unrealistic goals, not meeting the goals, and then feeling guilty so that you eat all the more and end up gaining weight, is devastating to your self-esteem. You need to deal with the problem realistically.

Learn to take small weight losses as positive steps to success. Isn't it better to lose one pound a week for thirty weeks and reach your goal weight than to lose ten pounds in one week and punish yourself so much in the process that you quit and regain all the weight you initially lost? In fact, if you are eating fewer than 1,200 calories, for a woman, or 1,500 calories, for a man, you may actually slow down your weight loss and compromise your health if you cut corners.

Now, take a few minutes to answer the questions in this self-study.

SELF-STUDY

1. Why do you want to lose weight?

2. Are there any reasons why you may *not* want to lose weight?

3. When you make a mistake and eat something which is not a healthy choice, are you able to admit the mistake and write it down?

4. Where in your home do you eat? List all locations.

5. Where do you eat when you are away from home? Do any of those places make it impossible for you to make wise food choices?

In James 5:7-8 we read, "See how the farmer waits for the land to yield its valuable crop and how patient he is for the autumn and spring rains. You too be patient and stand firm."

Losing weight is hard work and you need to be patient and stand firm in order to be successful. Your reward is a healthy body!

FIVE
Setting Your Goals

Most people have a goal weight in mind for themselves. Maybe you remember how much you weighed the last time you felt fit and looked good.

Maybe you failed the mirror test where you found those pounds you thought you had lost, or the "Can you pinch an inch?" test, or the belt test when you gasped for air as you tried to button the waist of your favorite pair of jeans.

Despite decades of research, experts have yet to find a reliable method of evaluating weight. We are all familiar with weight charts. Although they are good to use as a guideline, the problem is that the charts indicate an ideal or desirable weight but cannot tell the average person what percentage of that weight is from fat.

Many people with desirable weights may actually be obese. How can some "Skinny Minnie" be obese, you ask? Because obesity is a condition which exists when a person has more than the average percentage of fat to body weight. Men should have about 20 percent fat to body weight and women about 30 percent. Unfortunately, body weight and fat percentage are not the same. For example, during World War II, some military recruiters were embarrassed to learn that they had rejected some famous football players because they were overweight, when actually they had hardly any fat on their muscular bodies.

Using the Goal Weight Chart

You will find a Goal Weight Chart at the end of this chapter. The Goal Weight Chart is to be used as follows:

☐ Note the weight range for your height, sex, and frame size.

☐ Set a *temporary* goal weight which is five to fifteen pounds higher than the upper weight in your range.

☐ When you have reached this temporary goal weight, evaluate your weight loss record and, with the help of your doctor or a registered dietitian, set a permanent goal weight which is appropriate for you.

It is not possible to set an exact weight for yourself before you start to lose weight. People differ in body proportion of bone and muscle. If you have more than average of either, your desirable weight may be higher. If you have any doubt about what you should weigh or about your frame size, consult your doctor.

Graphing Your Weight Loss

Once you have established your goal weight, it is a good idea to start a graph which you can use to keep your weight in a lifetime perspective. It will teach you some important lessons about weight control. You may want to use the graph included at the end of this chapter. Or you can design your own.

Put your beginning weight in the upper left-hand corner of the graph. Along the left side of the graph, indicate the weight you will be losing in one-pound, five-pound, or ten-pound increments, depending on the amount of weight you have to lose. For example, if your beginning weight is 210 pounds, you would put 210 in the top left-hand corner and then put 209, 208, 207, 206, and so on, down the left side of the graph.

Figuring an average, sensible weight loss of one to one and one-half pounds per week, calculate the number of weeks it will take you to reach your temporary goal. For instance, if your beginning weight is 210 pounds and your temporary goal weight is 175 pounds, at one and one-half pounds per week it would take you twenty-three weeks to lose the thirty-five pounds. Put a dot at the point on the graph where the number of weeks to reach your temporary goal weight intersects with the weight at which you will be when you have reached your temporary goal weight. In our example, the person would put a dot where 175 pounds intersects with twenty-three weeks.

Draw a very light line between your beginning weight and the weight at which you plan to be in the number of weeks you have calculated it would take to reach your temporary goal.

Weigh Once a Week

On the same day of every week, only once a week, at the same time of day, wearing the same type of clothing, weighing on the same scale, record your weight loss on your chart by putting a dot beside the number of pounds you lost in the column for the current week. Going to a support group or sharing weight losses with a relative or friend can help to build your motivation to persevere.

Your actual experience is going to differ from the perfect line on your chart. This is true for everyone. Our bodies are not perfect machines and they respond with irregularity.

You may find that you lost more than one and one-half pounds per week the first two or three weeks on the program. Why such large losses? Won't you lose too much muscle tissue? This loss may be explained by the fact that you cut back your intake of calories and carbohydrates. Our bodies store excess carbohydrates in a large amount of fluid. When the extra calories are no longer consumed, the water which was used to store the old supply of carbohydrates is voided by the body. Since water weighs 8.2 pounds per gallon, this explains the rapid and encouraging weight loss many people experience in the first days of their weight loss program. It also explains why you may be spending more time in the bathroom the first few days. Do not blame it on drinking the water required by the *Weigh to Win* Rainbow Food Plan. Just realize that you are eating fewer calories and your body has to do something with the extra fluid in which the carbohydrates were stored.

Reasons for Inconsistent Weight Loss

Our bodies seldom lose weight consistently, even if we eat the same number of calories each day. There are several reasons for this fluctuation:

☐ All foods contain at least trace amounts of salt. On some days the sodium content of the foods we eat is higher than on other days. Salt leads to retention of fluids. Therefore, more salt means more liquid, which means more weight.

☐ Women fluctuate often because of their monthly cycles.

☐ Any change in activity can cause fluctuations in weight loss.

Any gains in weight which are caused by salt intake will be lost when the salt and the resulting fluid retention work their way out of your system. This might take a matter of weeks. I know that if I eat a piece of cured ham, the next morning I weigh three to four pounds more due to water retention from the salty meat. Sometimes it takes days or weeks before the scale goes back down.

At one time or another, despite the fact that we have been following our weight loss program "to the letter," many of us find that the scale just does not register a weight loss for a few weeks. Our weight may even increase somewhat. That is because the scale cannot tell the difference between fat and fluid. Eventually the fluids will be gone and the weeks of hard work will pay off. If you are on a plateau like this, it is critical that you keep careful track of what you eat on a Weekly Food Record. If you have not lost weight in a number of weeks, show your Weekly Food Records to your support group leader, family member, or close friend. They may be able to spot some problem foods such as ham, smoked turkey products, dill pickles, or salted popcorn which may lead to water retention. The Weekly Food Records will also be helpful to your doctor or registered dietitian if the problem is persistent.

New medications or changes in existing medications sometimes cause temporary fluid retention problems. Women on hormone therapy sometimes experience irregular weight loss due to fluid retention. If the plateau in weight loss is due to a decrease in activity, the body is left with extra calories that can be dealt with only by converting them to fat.

Those of us who are working hard to lose or maintain our weight are very sensitive to numbers on a scale. A plateau or even a small gain can cause discouragement, and then we decide that the weight loss plan just does not work. It is important that you not turn this into a catastrophe and decide that "all is lost" because of fluid retention or possibly because of a slight overindulgence.

You Overate and Still Lost Weight?

It is possible for weight loss to occur during a week in which overeating has taken place. This is when the deceiver devil comes in and tries to tell us, "See, you don't have to follow that silly food plan so closely to lose weight!" Or, more literally, "See, you can have your cake and eat it too!" Unfortunately, this thinking often leads to dramatic and disappointing weight loss failures.

If you overate and still managed to lose weight, it should be considered a temporary and unearned parole, not a reprieve. It is more important to analyze what caused the overeating and work on steps to develop better self-control in the future.

When you have not lost weight, despite the fact that there has been no overeating during the week, you should remind yourself that fat is being burned as long as food intake is reduced (yet kept to a healthy level) and activity levels are maintained or increased. You probably can expect a larger than normal weight loss in a few weeks as long as you do not deviate from the *Weigh to Win* Rainbow Food Plan.

Looking at your chart over the next weeks and months you will see peaks and valleys, but overall you should see progress that develops even higher levels of self-control.

Looking Ahead to Maintenance

Now let us do some looking ahead. Once you have reached your temporary goal weight, visit your doctor or registered dietitian and determine a final goal weight. Once again extend your chart to determine the number of weeks it will take to reach your final goal. When you have reached this joyful occasion you enter a new phase of your weight management program — maintenance.

You realize that your weight gains in the past were about one pound at a time, although you would have liked to think that you suddenly woke up one bleak morning twenty pounds heavier than when you went to bed.

If you are going to succeed at maintaining your weight loss, you will need to do the following:

☐ Keep accountable. Continue a weekly weigh-in with your support group, family member, or friend who has supported you through your weight loss.

☐ Permit yourself a very narrow channel of weight fluctuation. Do not ignore the problem. *Maintainers* take action when their weight is two to five pounds above goal. *Regainers* do not believe it is time for action until their weight has risen fifteen pounds or more. In the time it takes to gain back fifteen pounds, many bad habits could be strongly reestablished. It is vitally important that you add a warning bell to your chart once you reach your final goal. Put a dotted line from two to five pounds higher than your final goal weight and let this be a signal to you to work harder at self-control.

Perseverance and Patience

One of the most crucial elements of any weight loss effort is perseverance and patience. James 5:11 says, "As you know, we consider blessed those who have persevered. You have heard of Job's perseverance and have seen what the Lord finally brought about. The Lord is full of compassion and mercy." If you will persevere in your weight loss efforts, you and the Lord will bring about a trimmer, healthier you!

An important element of your successful weight loss is action. First Peter 1:13 states, "Therefore, prepare your minds for action; be self-controlled; set your hope fully on the grace to be given to you when Jesus Christ is revealed." You need to prepare your mind and be willing to change old habits which have caused you to overeat. Do not be afraid to take action and make better choices for your life.

Goal Weight Chart for Women

Height Feet	Inches	Small Frame	Medium Frame	Large Frame
4	10	102–111	109–121	118–131
4	11	103–113	111–123	120–134
5	0	104–115	113–126	122–137
5	1	106–118	115–129	125–140
5	2	108–121	118–132	128–143
5	3	111–124	121–135	131–147
5	4	114–127	124–138	134–151
5	5	117–130	127–141	137–155
5	6	120–133	130–144	140–159
5	7	123–136	133–147	143–163
5	8	126–139	136–150	146–167
5	9	129–142	139–153	149–170
5	10	132–145	142–156	152–173
5	11	135–148	145–159	155–176
6	0	138–151	148–162	158–179

Weights are for ages fifteen years and up. Weight is listed by pounds according to frame size (in indoor clothing weighing three pounds and shoes with a one-inch heel).

Goal Weight Chart for Men

Height Feet	Inches	Small Frame	Medium Frame	Large Frame
5	2	128–134	131–141	138–150
5	3	130–136	133–143	140–153
5	4	132–138	135–145	142–156
5	5	134–140	137–148	144–160
5	6	136–142	139–151	146–164
5	7	138–145	142–154	149–168
5	8	140–148	145–157	152–172
5	9	142–151	148–160	155–176
5	10	144–154	151–163	158–180
5	11	146–157	154–166	161–184
6	0	149–160	157–170	164–188
6	1	152–164	160–174	168–192
6	2	155–168	164–178	172–197
6	3	158–172	167–182	176–202
6	4	162–176	171–187	181–207

Children ten to fourteen years of age must have goal weights set by a physician.
If you have any questions about what you should weigh, please consult your physician.

Personal Weight Chart

Name _____

Height _____

Frame Size _____

Goal Weight Range _____

Beginning
Weight

Pounds in 1, 5, or 10 pound increments

NUMBER OF WEEKS

1 2 3 4 5 6 7 8 9 10 11 12 13 14 15 16 17 18 19 20 21 22 23 24 25 26 27 28 29 30 31 32 33 34 35 36 37 38 39 40 41 42 43 44 45 46 47 48 49 50 51 52

Six
Do Others Make You Eat?

"I am trying so hard," Meg said, "but Jim plops down after dinner to watch TV and makes me fix him a bowl of ice cream. He knows that I am trying to lose weight. He is always criticizing me about my weight and yet he says, 'Aw, come on, Meg—why don't you have some ice cream too—a little won't hurt you.' I don't know what to do. I can't seem to please him. The harder I try to lose weight, the harder Jim tries to keep me from succeeding."

"Mom tells me she loves me just as I am," cries thirteen-year-old Karen, who is 180 pounds, "and yet when we are in the mall, she goes to the petite section of the store and tells me how pretty I would look in a smaller size. Then, on the way home, Mom buys me an ice cream cone as a reward for having lost weight this week."

"Jerry bugged me constantly about my weight so I joined a *Weigh to Win* support group a friend of mine told me about. He knows my meeting is every Monday night and yet he makes plans for us almost every week and gets upset if I don't go along with him," sighs Verona.

"Howard is a workaholic and I never see him before 9 o'clock in the evening," Beth shrugs. "Since I've started going to a *Weigh to Win* support group, every Thursday he is home at 5:30 in the evening and says, 'You are always griping that I am never home, but here I am. I have made a special effort to come home and spend some time with you, and all you want to do is go off and be with those people at that fat club.' I just don't know what to do. He makes me feel so guilty."

Sarah's mother knew she was trying to lose weight but asked Sarah to come over for a special lunch. She arrived to find fried chicken, mashed potatoes laced with sour cream and cheese, creamed peas, and french silk pie for dessert—all foods which used to be her favorite dishes. When Sarah expressed dismay, her mother became upset and cried, "I just did it because I love you!"

Tom and Stan had been best friends for thirty years. Both had been overweight since childhood. When Tom started losing weight, Stan pulled away. The two used to bowl every week, but now Stan "had plans." At church, Tom was getting a lot of compliments about his weight loss. Stan was asked, "When are you going to lose weight too?" Stan had a five-pound box of sausage and cheese sent to Tom's house for Easter.

"George was so encouraging through my weight loss; but now that I have almost reached my goal weight, he is questioning everything I do. He always wants to know where I am going and how long I will be gone. If I'm gone any longer, he gives me the third degree about who I was with. I even caught him checking the mileage on my car to see if I was telling the truth about where I went. When I was fat,

George never acted this way. I find myself wanting to eat and get fat again, just so he will quit this insane jealousy." Marie closed her eyes tightly to hold back the tears.

Then there is the family member who refuses to eat out anywhere except places where there are few healthy choices to be made; the spouse who complains that there is "never anything good to eat in this house anymore"; or the children who refuse to even taste any new dish just because they think it is "diet food."

Passing the Pizza

I was fortunate in that my family was very supportive throughout my weight loss and in the years since. It was, however, a learning process for all of us. Sometimes, especially at the beginning of my weight loss, my teenage children would ask for a pizza for supper. I would tell myself that I could "handle it" and put together a quick healthy meal just for me before the pizza arrived. Invariably, the pizza was harder to resist than I thought. I remember watching the pizza box being passed back and forth across the table and right in front of my nose. When I reached for the box, my children started a game of "keep away," tossing the pizza over my head and out of my reach all the time quoting, "Nothing tastes as good as being thin feels!"

Another time, I actually got my hands on a piece of pizza. I quickly shut the box. No one said anything as I ate the whole piece. I opened the box a second time and started for a second piece. My husband said, "How much of that are you going to eat?" I said, "Quite possibly the whole thing." Then he said, "No, you're not—I need it for my lunch tomorrow," closed the box and put it in the refrigerator, saving me from disaster.

Weight Loss With or Without Family Support

Through my years of teaching *Weigh to Win* classes, I was quickly made aware that a great number of people do not have the support I experienced with my family. My heart ached as I heard one story after another of the difficulties many people experience with family and close friends as they try to lose weight. *Weigh to Win* members pleaded with me to address the issue in our support group lessons.

I went to see a Christian psychologist about the subject and was amazed to learn that he saw four to five people a week who sought counseling because of the battles they faced when they tried to lose weight. Further research revealed more and more of the tragedy that class members have been expressing to me through the years. Why does this happen? What makes a husband, wife, parent, brother, sister, or close friend suddenly change when we make an effort to lose weight?

Impacters Make an Impact on You

There are all kinds of psychological names for the people we have been describing, such as *codependents* and *enablers*. I prefer to call persons who take action, whether directly or indirectly, to make it difficult for you to lose weight and maintain your weight loss, *impacters*. Impacters seek to undermine or destroy your weight loss effort for reasons which, consciously or subconsciously, are selfish. Whatever the reason, the actions of the impacter have an impact on you!

Why does the impacter behave in this way? When we lose weight, especially large amounts of weight, there is a kind of renewal that takes place which has its own impact on those closest to us. I could feel myself changing mentally, physically, and spiritually as I lost weight. I had a new confidence in myself which had not been there before. Instead of just wanting to go home after church each Sunday, I wanted to get together with some new people and get to know them over a nice meal in a restaurant. My husband loves to socialize, so he really enjoyed this change. However, many husbands enjoy coming home, sitting down to read the Sunday paper, and taking a "Sunday snooze." What an upsetting change when, all of a sudden, his wife wants to go out to dinner every week.

I had not been the kind to want to go shopping, because buying clothes in my size had been such a chore and an embarrassment. As I lost more and more weight, I loved finding out I could fit into a smaller size. I begged my husband to come along and promised him I would give him a "fashion show" if he would help me decide which clothes looked best. Buying new clothes was not easy on our budget, but my husband was so proud of me that he would just say, "You keep losing weight, and we will find a way to get clothes for you." I wore a lot of hand-me-downs and shopped at resale shops too. When you lose as much weight as I did, *everything* changes sizes—shoes, underwear—even my watch had to have links taken out of it.

If my husband had been an impacter, he would have griped about every new piece of clothing. Instead of sharing my happiness about getting into smaller sizes, he would have criticized and belittled, saying things like, "Why spend the money? You will just gain all the weight back and won't be able to wear it anyway," or "Who are you buying those new things for?"

Weight Loss Brings a Spiritual Change

I changed spiritually too. Although I knew the Lord loved me as I was before, I now felt I could come to Him with more confidence because I was changing bad eating habits into good healthy choices daily. I was taking care of my body, God's temple, and my joy overflowed into my spiritual life. I wanted to find what the Lord's will was for my life, and I had the confidence and assurance from Him to do just that. I felt the Lord leading me to help others lose weight as I had, and this started my ministry with overweight people through *Weigh to Win.* I talked with my husband about the doors that were opening to begin this ministry and what it might mean. We would have people in our home every week for class, and some would call for help at all hours of the day and night. I might have to be gone in the evening teaching other classes. Speaking tours would mean extended absences from home. My husband and family all said, "Go for it!" Everybody in the family pitched in to help.

In a few months I had to give up my full-time job, but instead of complaining, my husband just tried to build up his bread route to help make up for our loss in income (he had left the full-time pastorate when we moved back to Indiana). My mother ran copies of my materials, and the children spent their Christmas vacation assembling 100,000 pages of cookbooks. If there had been an impacter in my house, the reaction would probably have been, "What do you know about starting your own business?" or "Do you have to be gone again? I came home especially early to see you."

My husband and family enjoyed watching my happiness grow. Sure, there were a lot of changes. They had to learn to eat some foods they had never eaten before. And if they ate a candy bar, they had better not leave any evidence of it in the house! But, instead of complaining, my family gave support, encouragement, and cooperation.

One time I heard my daughter calling across the school auditorium to a friend, "Gina, Gina, come here! You've just got to see my mom!" She was so proud of my weight loss that she had to show me off.

Would I have succeeded had there been an impacter in my house? I don't know, but if I had, I do know it would have been much harder. In order for the *Weigh to Win* ministry to become more helpful to those who live with an impacter, I realized I must learn more about impacters and their motivation.

As I was researching this subject and talking to my husband about it, he surprised me by revealing some deep feelings. While I was losing weight, I was working in the office of an industrial manufacturing plant. As I got close to my goal weight, I became aware that the men in the plant began to treat me differently. They would come up and linger around my desk or would hurry to open a door. A company executive even grabbed me in the coffee room and gave me a "friendly" hug. This was all very disconcerting to me. I was not behaving any differently than before my weight loss. I am "true blue" to my husband and would never think of being unfaithful; but learning how to handle these men was a new experience and, I will admit, somewhat flattering at first. When I was overweight, no one rushed to open a door for me even if my arms were full of packages.

I would go home and share these experiences with my husband because we can talk about everything. I just laughed them off and didn't even notice that my husband was not laughing.

When we began to talk about the subject of impacters, he revealed how he had felt when I told him about the change in behavior from the men at the plant. He shared that some of his insecurities and fears started coming to the surface. He began to think, "Lynn sees me with all my faults and weaknesses. Having pastored small churches for ten years, I have never been able to give her a lot of things materially. What if some 'knight in shining armor' comes along who is more handsome and has a lot of money? Perhaps he could do all the things I am not very good at, like fixing things around the house and balancing a checkbook. I could possibly lose the woman I love!"

I had no idea my husband felt this way. In my mind, there was no doubt that I loved him with all my heart and that there would never be anyone else for me, even if I did see all of his "warts." I knew he had to live with all of my faults and weaknesses too and still love me. Yet, if those feelings were there in a marriage as good as ours, how much stronger might they be in a marriage which teetered on a weak foundation?

Why Do Impacters Behave as They Do?

Impacters behave out of fear. It is a fear that as you change, gain confidence, and improve yourself mentally, physically, and spiritually, their own weaknesses and insecurities will seem magnified. Fear is especially hard for men to deal with because it is considered a weakness. Anger, however, is a strong emotion and considered more acceptable for men. Therefore, their fear gets translated into anger. Instead of saying, "You look so beautiful that I am afraid some other man will sweep you off your feet and I will lose you," an impacter will turn that fear to anger with words like, "You may think I don't know, but I know where you have been and who you have been with—don't lie to me!"

Your weight loss makes the impacters have to face their own shortcomings. If they get a glimpse of these and choose not to change, then their only option is for things to stay the way they were, and that means keeping you overweight. Change is harder for some people than for others. In the time it takes you to lose weight, a lot of renegotiation of your relationships needs to take place.

Will Your Relationship Survive?

Relationships will survive this transition if they have a good foundation. If you are in a relationship with an impacter, it is a symptom of a problem more serious than the fact that you are losing weight—it indicates a weak foundation. When the impacter reacts in anger, he is really saying,

☐ "I am surprised you love me."

☐ "As long as you are fat, I don't have to worry about anyone else taking you away from me."

☐ "When you are fat you don't feel good about yourself, so you are dependent on me and that is the way I like it."

☐ "If you look better, you won't need me anymore."

Impacters are not able to articulate these subconscious feelings, and so they express their fears by criticizing, complaining, and belittling. Impacters are subconsciously trying to make you feel so guilty that you will slack off. If they can get you to miss just one support group meeting or eat one bowl of ice cream, then the foot is in the door to get you to miss other meetings or make other poor food choices, and they will make every effort to see that you do so.

As a Christian, you may also be faced with the thought that if you are trying to do something to make yourself look better, then you are being selfish. All the vanity verses come to mind. Impacters will use these Scriptures and these fears to their advantage, making you feel that if you go to a support group meeting you are neglecting your family and therefore sinning. Their focus is not on how this weight loss will improve your health, but on how selfish and vain you are. You need to remind yourself that you may have become overweight because you have not felt good about yourself.

Impacters work to keep you dependent because they are afraid of losing their identity. Subconsciously, your positive changes make them take a look at themselves and they are afraid to try to be any different.

If you have an impacter in your life, there are two options available to you. You can let this person make you feel guilty and self-centered, and then give up on your weight loss efforts. This will certainly make peace and let the impacter know he has won. But how will you feel about yourself? What are you likely to do as a response to these feelings? What have you done in the past? Have you turned to food?

Your other option is to stand your ground. You are taking a risk in doing this. The relationship will either crumble, or your firmness will force the impacter to take a look at himself and face his own insecurities. Hopefully, he too will grow from the process. Both of you could come through the change as better, more confident people who allow each other the space to grow and improve.

When my husband began to confront some of the insecurities he had been feeling, instead of taking them out on me as an impacter would have, he worked on his own weight loss and lost thirty pounds. He even started coming to class to weigh in each week. He suggested we buy matching mountain bikes, and we had fun taking a biking vacation around the north shore of Lake Superior. He began going on walks with me. Not only did these changes help him physically, but they also drew us closer together. We shared more activities because we both wanted to work on being physically fit.

Change always involves risk, and so it is with close relationships. Some of us take the necessary risks and give each other space, encouragement, and support as we grow and experience life together. Others of us are not secure enough in ourselves to take risks, and so we tend to hinder the other's efforts toward growth, independence, and wholeness.

In any relationship, we should want the best for each other. But what do we mean by "best"? Sometimes the word gets distorted as our own feelings of insecurity weave their way into the situation.

If the relationship is to grow stronger through the years, we need to make some choices. A good foundation is built by two people who listen to each other's feelings and opinions and then find ways to express caring and support, to encourage each other, not to tear each other down. They develop attitudes that allow them both to reach their full potential and be all that God would have them to be.

Fear causes us to keep people we love from becoming whole and happy. Pride keeps us from admitting our fears. A mixture of fear and pride keeps us from expressing our mutual insecurities, because we are afraid of losing the love of the other person.

If you are in a relationship with an impacter, you will have to work hard at both your relationship *and* losing weight. Can it be done? I have seen many dear people in just such a relationship succeed at their weight loss with the help of the Lord. In some instances, the relationship survived and improved. In most, the relationship did not change, but the *Weigh to Win* member developed coping skills to succeed, despite the odds. In a few cases, the relationship did not continue. Philippians 2:1-5 gives the pattern for a good relationship:

> If you have any encouragement from being united with Christ, if any comfort from His love, if any fellowship with the Spirit, if any tenderness and compassion, then make my joy complete by being like-minded, having the

same love, being one in spirit and purpose. Do nothing out of selfish ambition or vain conceit, but in humility consider others better than yourselves. Each of you should look not only to your own interests, but also to the interests of others. Your attitude should be the same as that of Christ Jesus.

Love is not meant to negatively impact others. Loving someone means supporting them and helping them reach their full potential. This kind of relationship means each partner is happier as a person and as a partner.

If you are in a relationship similar to the ones we have shared in this chapter, I urge you to consider talking to a professional Christian counselor or pastor. My prayers are with you.

SEVEN

Learning to Make Wise Food Choices

How do we learn to reach for the carrot instead of the candy bar? What makes us want the apple—not the apple pie? How do we keep our eyes from automatically scanning the dessert section first on the restaurant menu? Just as we have learned to make poor food choices or to overeat, so now we have to learn to make healthy food choices on a daily basis.

Do Not "Diet"

The learning process begins with changing our thoughts about eating correctly. It is important not to think of the *Weigh to Win Weight Management System* as "going on a diet." Diets automatically trigger a negative response in most people. To those of us who have tried everything to lose weight, a "diet" means deprivation and hunger. A "diet" means eating monotonous, tasteless foods. A "diet" means drinking diet milk shakes which seem to have sand in the bottom. A "diet" means going to a party and not being able to eat anything. A "diet" means failure. A "diet" means crushed self-esteem.

Instead of dieting, concentrate on feeding your body foods

which the Lord created, in the amounts that He meant for your body to consume. Concentrate on all the wonderful choices you *can* have, and begin to unravel the cords that pull you to the foods you have craved in the past.

Accurate Nutritional Information Is Essential

To learn to make wise food choices, we need accurate nutritional information so that we are not swayed by the marketing schemes of some food producers. We are constantly bombarded with new "diet" or "lite" products which come on the market. Often these are just watered-down versions of the original. Many bakeries are producing fat-free cakes and donuts which sound like a waist watcher's dream. But when we check the amount of sugar in the product, we see something quite different. Such products often cause confusion and complicate attempts to make healthy choices.

Making wise food choices involves learning how new nutritional information fits into your way of life, learning how to make nutrition work with your personality, and then eliminating the excuses you often use to avoid making the needed changes in diet.

Keeping It Simple

I am a detail person. I can take a confused mess and organize it in a short time. However, when it comes to feeding my body, I have learned the K.I.S.S. method which is "Keep It Simple, Stupid." This is something I have to tell myself from time to time to jolt me to attention. When I try to get too complicated with my food choices, shopping, and preparation, it usually means trouble.

Previous attempts to lose weight began with five weeks of menu plans complete with several new recipes to try each week. Of course, the grocery list was all planned out. I would even organize the list to group like foods together, to make my shopping more efficient and to keep from going down aisles which should be avoided (like the potato chip and candy aisles). This organization caused just a few problems. If a certain food on my list was not available, sold out, or of poor quality, it threw me into a real dither. Why, without that particular food the meal I had planned was ruined. If that meal was ruined, then the whole day's meal plans were messed up. If the day was a disaster, the whole week must be terrible. I would give up in frustration and buy a bag of cookies.

Then there were the days when I was just too tired to cook the elaborate meal I had planned, or when we were invited to someone's home for dinner. Each event spelled disaster for my weight loss plans. I was completely rigid. The program I was trying to follow had no flexibility built in—it was not livable.

As I was developing the *Weigh to Win* Rainbow Food Plan, I realized I needed to avoid overcomplicating my life and setting myself up for failure. All the intricate organization had just given me excuses to fail. How could I simplify my eating so that I had no reason to fail?

Stock the Refrigerator with Healthy Foods

The first step is to *keep the refrigerator stocked with healthy foods*. I do not mean a stockpile of bulgur, leeks, and brewer's yeast. Remember, my new motto was simplicity, and shopping at a health food store did not fit into my hectic life. Now I shop with a simplified grocery list. I head right for the produce aisle and stock up on a variety of fruits and vegetables.

I used to buy a bag of oranges and a bag of apples. Half of

them would rot before they were eaten. You see, I knew what I should be eating, but why eat an apple when there was a package of cheese Danishes in the bread box? I have learned to choose smaller amounts of many kinds of fruit. Why just buy one kind of lettuce when there are so many tastes, textures, and colors available? My refrigerator looks like a rainbow of colors after going grocery shopping. Since I dislike cleaning vegetables, I make myself do the chore as I am putting away the groceries so that the job is all done at once. Otherwise, having to clean vegetables becomes an excuse to eat a food which is not a wise choice.

Keeping a variety of canned vegetables on hand makes it easy to just warm up a vegetable rather than having to cook fresh or frozen vegetables for those "in a hurry" times. Sliced breast of turkey makes a quick sandwich eaten cold or a nice entree when warmed in the microwave. The in-store delicatessens will even weigh small portions for you so that you can be sure of the size. Cottage cheese, peanut butter, an occasional egg, and sliced cheese are all ready-made sources of protein.

Sugar-free and nonfat yogurts make a good treat and are a healthy choice. Sugar-free hot cocoa mixes and sugar-free instant puddings help to provide the calcium needed each day, and they are so delicious that there is no reason to feel deprived. Best of all, they are ready in seconds. I can whip up a batch of chocolate pudding much faster than it takes to bake a cake mix.

Enriched white bread is not an unhealthy choice, but whole grain breads and cereals add fiber to your daily food intake, making your body function more efficiently. My German heritage is an advantage in this area. My family says I eat "gravel bread" because the chewier, heavier, and darker the bread is, the more I enjoy it.

It is helpful to buy several turkeys when they are on sale

during the holidays. You do not have to bother stuffing them. If you cut the turkeys into quarters, they bake faster and are easier to handle. Remove all visible fat, skin, and bones. Weigh the meat and divide it into a variety of individual and family portions. Cooked turkey stored in your freezer means your entree just needs to be warmed and you are ready to go.

Do you enjoy brown rice but do not like how long it takes to fix? Make up a double or triple batch at a time and then before you are tempted to eat more than you should, divide the rice into portions and freeze. *Voila!* Instant rice whenever you need it.

Just because I like to eat "gravel bread," brown rice, and yogurt does not mean that you have to eat these foods, if you do not like them. I do encourage you to be open to trying new foods or some you may not have tried in a long time. Tastes do change. You may be surprised to find that you like a food which you used to avoid. The guiding principle is to stock your refrigerator with healthy foods which are enjoyable and easy to prepare.

Trying an occasional new recipe adds variety and interest to your choices. Do not eat the same foods every day. I once overheard a support group member comment how tired she was of eating open-faced tuna sandwiches every day for lunch. With all the variety of healthy foods available, there is no reason for such monotony. Never get into the same-food-everyday rut just to avoid thinking about what to prepare! You will set yourself up for sure failure. God put a *variety* of foods on this earth for us to enjoy.

Write Down What You Eat

Now that you have your refrigerator stocked with a colorful rainbow of foods, what is going to keep you from sending your spouse out for a carton of ice cream when you feel like a binge? The second step is to *write down every morsel you eat just before you eat it*. Keeping a Food Record keeps you accountable. How many times have you forgotten by evening what you ate for breakfast? Do not rely on your memory.

By recording your food intake, you can be certain to consume all of the foods necessary to meet your body's daily nutritional needs. If you do not write down what you eat, you may end up eating too much from one food group and too little from another. You may find yourself craving food to satisfy the nutritional deficit. It becomes too easy to reach for the foods to which you have habitually turned in order to satisfy food cravings, instead of stopping to analyze what you should eat in order to achieve the balance of foods your body needs each day.

The Weekly Food Records available with the *Weigh to Win Weight Management System* make it easy to keep track of your food intake on a daily and weekly basis. To help keep yourself accountable, make a pact to exchange Food Records with a friend, relative, or a support group member each week. Be completely honest and write down everything you eat. You cannot help another person unless you are honest with yourself first. In Job 31:4 and 6 we read, "Does He not see my ways and count my every step? . . . Let God weigh me in honest scales and He will know that I am blameless."

If you made a poor choice of foods, the discipline of writing it down on your Food Record is not a reason to kick yourself for the rest of the week and feel guilty about what you did. Challenge yourself to learn from your mistake. Analyze why you made the choice at that time. Was the choice triggered by an emotion, an event, or a situation with which you have learned to associate food in the past?

Instead of dwelling on the mistake, congratulate yourself on all the times you successfully made healthy choices and ate well. Always build on your successes, instead of getting mired down with defeat.

"Yagottawanna"

Step three is "yagottawanna." No weight loss program will work for you unless you want to change. The *Weigh to Win Weight Management System* gives you an easy road map toward healthful eating, but you have to take the journey. I cannot be there to take food out of your hands or put good healthy food into your body. "You gotta want to!"

The desire to change does not have to be a strong feeling. The desire to have a better quality of life by learning to eat well may start as just a small seed of resolve. Resolve means doing what you know you have to do to achieve a worthwhile goal or purpose. Resolve often begins as something very small, just like the biblical mustard plant, "I tell you the truth, if you have faith as small as a mustard seed . . . nothing will be impossible for you" (Matthew 17:20). Resolve grows as we proceed through this new way of eating one day at a time, and as those habits which once controlled us begin to be controlled *by* us.

Ask the Lord for His Help

Step four is to *ask the Lord for strength and wisdom.* I was seated next to a woman on a flight from Seattle to Chicago. I enjoy getting to know new people on my travels and, in the course of conversation, the "What type of work do you do?" question usually comes up. I am always ready and willing to talk about *Weigh to Win* and my weight loss. It seems that usually I am seated next to someone with a weight problem. Since some 65 million Americans are overweight, the odds of this happening are in my favor.

As we learned more about each other, this lovely woman quietly said, "I never thought of asking God to help me with my weight problem." I have heard other people say this, and the thought always surprises me because I was just the opposite. I begged the Lord to take away all my fat. I begged Him to keep me from eating. I begged Him to remove all of the tempting foods on the earth. I would cry and plead with Him to take away my desire to overeat. Of course, He did not answer my prayers, because I was not taking responsibility for the choices I was making or admitting that I had to do my part.

"My grace is sufficient for you, for My power is made perfect in weakness" (2 Corinthians 12:9).

The Lord knows our weaknesses, and while He is not going to supernaturally remove our desire for foods we shouldn't eat, He does promise that His grace is sufficient for us.

If we tell Him that it is our desire to make healthful choices of foods instead of eating the way we have learned to eat in the past, He will be there to give us the strength we need to resist. Do you understand what I am saying? God will not keep us from overeating but, if we show Him that it is our heart's desire to make better choices, He promises that His power will overcome our weakness.

You do not have to be strong and highly motivated to be successful with your weight loss. All you need is the Lord and a small seed of resolve to get you started. Take one step at a time. God will be with you, and I will be praying for you.

Proverbs 21:20 says, "In the house of the wise are stores of choice food." Pray for the Lord's guidance that you will learn to keep stores of *choice* food in your home and that you will be able to make the best *choices* every day.

EIGHT

The Formula for Successful Weight Loss

On paper, the formula for successful weight loss seems quite simple. Weight is *maintained* when the body takes in just enough energy in the form of food to keep its vital processes going and its muscles active. Weight is *gained* when more energy is taken in than is needed for these two purposes. Weight is *lost* when energy consumption falls below energy need. In other words, weight is simply a product of supply and demand. When the supply and demand of energy are in balance, weight is maintained. When supply exceeds demand, weight is gained; and when demand is greater than supply, weight is lost.

When we take in more food energy than we need at the moment, our bodies burn what they need and store most of the rest. Later, if energy output exceeds intake, our bodies turn to those stores and burn up some of their supply. When we store extra energy for future needs, we do to ourselves the same thing that we do to our cars when we put gas in the tank. The average gas tank holds enough fuel to allow the car to cruise from 200–400 miles between filling stations. If the car's gas tank were enlarged so that it could hold 200 gallons instead of 20 gallons, it might have a greater cruising range;

however, 20 gallons of gas weighs under 200 pounds and 200 gallons weighs close to 2,000 pounds. What do you think would happen to your car with this much added weight on it? The frame would have to be built more sturdily. The tires would have to be enlarged, and it would certainly burn a lot more gasoline. Do you ever feel as if your body is getting fewer miles to the gallon? Do you eat and eat but still have little energy for normal activities? You normally store enough food energy for five or six days of life. If you add to your supplies enough for fifty or sixty days, you put a strain on your bone structure and joints and reduce your mobility. In addition, you get sharply reduced mileage (energy) from the food you consume, because it takes an increased amount of food energy just to maintain a heavier body weight.

The energy balance equation is universal, but it does not apply equally to all people. Some overweight people eat far more than some thin people, as you can often observe in public eating places. But many others eat as little or even less than thin people, with the major difference being not how much energy goes in, but how much energy goes out in the form of physical activity.

Also, some people seem able to "waste" calories: they eat a lot, do little, and still do not gain very much weight. Other people are very efficient and, for them, every calorie counts. For all, however, the basic weight control formula is the same: to lose weight, cut intake relative to output.

How Our Bodies Store Energy

Our bodies store energy from the foods we eat in three different forms.

☐ Some energy is stored as *carbohydrates* in the bloodstream, muscles, and liver. Carbohydrates are actually glycogen and sugar, and are very important because they become an immediate, available fuel supply for the organs. At only four calories per gram, carbohydrates do not deserve their reputation as being fattening. Avoiding potatoes, breads, and pastas is not the answer to losing weight. Avoiding the high-fat sour cream, butter, sauces, and gravies which we put on the potatoes, breads, and pastas will keep you on the right track.

The Bible is filled with references to bread. Although the word *bread* was used as a general term for food or nourishment, there is no doubt about the importance of bread throughout the Scriptures. Jesus even referred to Himself as the "Bread of life" in John 6:35.

Simple carbohydrates in the form of manufactured sugars and honey add *empty calories* to your daily food intake. Empty calories come from foods which have little or no nutritive value; limit these foods as much as possible.

A feeling of lightheadedness can result when the body's supply of carbohydrates falls below the necessary life-supporting level. The body works hard to keep an adequate supply of glycogen or blood sugar at all times.

☐ Energy is also stored as *protein,* which is the building block of the body's muscles and organs. The body turns first to carbohydrates for an immediate source of energy, and then, if that supply is low, it begins to convert protein to energy. This conversion could seriously weaken the body, because tissue loss from any of its muscles, the heart, brain, liver, or other organs can impair its ability to survive. Protein is a poor source of fuel. It supplies only four calories of energy per gram. Because protein is about 80 percent water, one pound of it would net only 450 calories or about one-sixth of the daily energy need of a typical young man.

☐ *Fat* is the most concentrated of the body's fuel supplies. It yields nine calories per gram and, because fat is only 15 percent fluid, one pound of fat yields 3,500 calories. This is the critical number for all people concerned about losing weight because, within small variations, the average man or woman who takes in an extra 3,500 calories—over a period of hours, days, or weeks—gains close to one pound of fat, while the person who takes in 3,500 calories fewer than he or she burns—again over a period of hours, days, or weeks—will lose one pound of fat, give or take a little.

Let us look at a thirty-year-old woman who is five feet four inches tall and weighs 225 pounds. We can assume for the purpose of this illustration that she normally needs 2,600 calories to meet her body's daily energy needs. If she cuts her daily food intake to approximately 1,200 calories, eats a balanced diet from each of the food groups and maintains her usual level of activity, she will draw upon her energy reserves for 1,400 calories daily. This means that in two days she will burn up 2,800 calories more than her food intake. In three days this will amount to 4,200 calories worth, and so on. Every day that she takes in 1,400 calories fewer than her energy output demands, she could lose four-tenths of a pound. Although this loss will not register on the scale every day, in 250 days she will have lost 100 pounds and be at her goal weight of 125 pounds.

Because the body can do nothing with extra energy other than store it, taking in even a few extra calories every day can lead to a large weight gain. For example, eating one small seventy-calorie cookie in addition to your energy needs could lead to a gain of an extra pound of fat every seven weeks, or between seven and eight pounds per year. Carried over a period of four or five years, this very small indulgence can add up to a serious weight problem. I know that I gained much of my weight at a rate of about ten pounds a year, but in ten years that is 100 pounds!

Sometimes people remark, "But I only have 10 pounds to lose!" and I say to them, "Most of us wish we had taken care of the problem when we had just 10 pounds to lose, instead of 40 or 60 or 100 pounds."

Fortunately, I have some good news for you. The formula for gaining weight we just talked about works exactly the same way in reverse! Eliminating one cookie or about seventy calories from your daily diet, in conjunction with the nutritious *Weigh to Win* Rainbow Food Plan, can lead to a very satisfying weight loss at year's end.

Impatience Means Impossible

Because most of us are impatient, we are not happy with the idea of taking 250 days to achieve any goal, even one as important as losing weight. We try to speed up the process by taking pills with or without a doctor's prescription. We take laxatives or try to vomit away our binges. Or we try to eat as little as possible, often without medical supervision. There are three problems with all of these schemes.

☐ It is often either unhealthy or impossibly uncomfortable to follow them for long.

☐ During the process, no new constructive habits are learned. Therefore, maintaining the weight loss is all but impossible. Weight lost in a hurry is nearly always regained just about as fast.

☐ Rapid weight loss, if it leads to quick regains, can be bad for your health.

The Yo-Yo syndrome of fast weight loss and fast weight gain can be very bad for your health. Fat deposits build up in the bloodstream while weight is being gained, and there is little evidence that these deposits are lost when you lose weight again. The important thing is to begin a "fat conscious" lifestyle which will not increase these deposits.

Besides the possible health consequences, crushed self-esteem is another result of attempts to lose weight the "quick and easy" way. You will do well to avoid wonder diets, devices, and drugs which may have been promoted by people who claim to have discovered "nature's long-buried secret." What you need instead is a program which will lead to an average loss of from one-half to two pounds per week. Any program which brings you down too quickly is likely to bump you back up just as fast, and you will be much the worse for wear.

Diets of 1,200 to 1,400 calories per day for women, and 1,600 to 1,800 calories per day for men, are likely to offer the opportunity for just such a gradual loss of weight. The lower end of the calorie range would be best for you if you are less active or have a small frame size for your sex and height. You will need the higher end of the range if you are more active than most and if you have a larger frame size.

Characteristics of a Sound Weight Loss Program

A sound weight loss program must have these four important characteristics.

☐ It must provide all of your minimum daily food requirements.

☐ It must give you enough to eat so that you are not faced with constant hunger.

☐ It must give you enough variety every day so that your desire for different tastes and textures is satisfied.

☐ It must provide you with an education for lifelong changes in what you eat.

If the program you choose does not meet your body's daily nutritional needs, you may risk serious nutritional inadequacies which could impair your health. If you eat so little that you are always hungry, you are likely to quickly give up because your appetite will never rest. If you eat the same few foods day after day, the monotony will cause you to give up out of boredom. If the diet that you follow is eccentric because it gives you few choices or requires you to eat foods which are not normally available, you will have little chance of following the program in the years after your weight goal has been reached. The *Weigh to Win Weight Management System* meets these requirements—gradual weight loss, nutritional balance, prevention of hunger, satisfaction to your appetite, and maintenance for life. As you lose weight, if you do not reeducate yourself to choose foods wisely, you will have little hope of maintaining your weight loss.

View your weight-loss journey with the *Weigh to Win Weight Management System* as a time of personal and spiritual renewal. Eat all of the foods which are allowed, so that you feel satisfied and your body is properly nourished. Proverbs 22:12 says, "The eyes of the Lord keep watch over knowledge." Read and learn everything you can about nutrition, but be sure it is from reputable sources. Then, let the Lord teach you how to choose food wisely, while you strengthen your resolve with your successful weight loss.

NINE
What Are You Weighing?

When you step on the scale each week, have you thought about *what* you are weighing? Yes, I know you are weighing pounds, but you really are weighing much more than that.

You Weigh Your Attitudes

If you have had a positive attitude about learning to eat nutritiously, if you have had a positive attitude about yourself, if you have had a positive attitude about the healthy choices of foods you made, if you have had a positive attitude about recording your food intake daily on your Food Record, the scale will probably reflect these attitudes. (Sometimes our bodies hold water, and even the most positive attitude cannot make the scale tell the difference between fat and fluid. Overall, however, a healthy attitude will mean a good steady weight loss.)

You Weigh the Past

Poor eating habits learned in childhood and carried into adulthood are reflected on the scales because the person you are now is battling with those habits. When I was a child, we had Kool-Aid at almost every meal; sugar was sprinkled on sliced tomatoes, and was added to most dishes containing tomatoes or tomato sauce; sugar was added to corn and peas, and sprinkled on grapefruit; bread soaked in milk and coated with sugar was one of our favorite treats. I learned to like food that tasted sweet. It took a long while for me to learn to enjoy the real taste of food without added sugar.

My brothers and I would be chided for leaving food on our plates. We were taught to push down with the backs of our forks to get every crumb off of the plate. While we were only being taught what our parents had been taught, I had to realize that it was time the cycle be broken.

I practiced exercising control over my food by occasionally leaving a couple of green beans on my plate during my weight loss. I still test myself often to be sure I can leave a little food on my plate; otherwise, I know that the food, and my past, still can and will control me.

You Weigh How You Deal with the Past

If you were raised in a dysfunctional home where emotions were poorly handled, and where there may have been alcoholism, illegal drugs, sexual abuse, or domestic violence, you bring all that baggage with you to the scales. You can pray and leave your past in the Lord's hands, but you never really forget.

My great-grandmother used to say, "It is a crater when you are in it and a dimple when you are out." Even when the situation or circumstance is far behind us, the "dimple" remains when a particular incident, smell, person, or event brings a painful memory to mind.

Karen shared how her stepfather would sexually abuse her and then give her a piece of chocolate. Susan explained that after her mother had beaten her and the rage had subsided, her mother would buy her ice cream and beg her forgiveness. Janet's husband would beat her in an alcoholic rage and then order pizza to be delivered so that she would not have to cook. Each weekend Shelly was ordered by the court to stay with her father and stepmother. Her father was seldom home and the stepmother made her clean the entire house. If Shelly did a good job, she was given candy as a reward. These dear women were being taught that food was the answer to their problems. Now, whenever a problem develops, their immediate response is to turn to food.

Do you turn to food without even realizing it? The Lord can help to make you aware of your eating, if you will but ask. The Lord will watch out for us, "For the eyes of the Lord range throughout the earth to strengthen those whose hearts are fully committed to Him" (2 Chronicles 16:9).

Many times through my weight loss and even now, I know the Lord brings to mind an awareness of the choices I must make, and then gives me the strength to make the right choices if I will but ask Him.

Awareness is the first step in conquering any habit. I used to be in the bad habit of saying, "Ya' know." I could hardly say a single sentence without including this phrase. It had become such a habit that I did not even realize how much this commonly used slang expression had punctuated my speech. My mother helped me to break the habit, because every time I would say "Ya' know" she would say, "No, I don't know." Her comment would interrupt my sentence and break my concentration. However, once I realized what she was trying to do—to bring the problem to a level of my awareness—her interruption became the first step in conquering the habit. After all, if this little phrase annoyed her, it must have annoyed others who would not think of correcting me.

It took several weeks. Soon I began catching myself just as I said the phrase. After a while, I was able to catch myself before I actually said the phrase. Now, it is not a part of my speech, and I don't even think about it.

At first, developing an awareness of what you are eating, when you are eating, and why you are eating, consumes your thoughts, interferes with your daily activities, and puts a "kink" in your lifestyle. As the awareness grows, it can even become depressing when you realize how often you habitually turn to food. You begin to feel that you can never conquer the problem because it is there with you every waking moment.

You know that you are on the way to overcoming the habit when food no longer is on your mind most of the time. Instead of considering what you will have for lunch before breakfast is even over, you will find yourself not thinking about lunch until just before time to eat. This *will* happen. You *can* break the chains of your past. You *will* be able to eat the right amounts and for the right reasons.

Be patient with yourself. You did not learn these habits overnight and they will not disappear overnight. It is no wonder that Galatians 5:22 lists "patience" as one of the fruits of the Spirit.

You Weigh Your Emotions

If you had a stressful week and responded to it by turning to food, you weighed your stress. A young college student, who found himself munching on all the poor choices of foods found around college dorms, admitted that boredom was a problem for him. Are you lonely, and do you keep trying to fill up the hole left by the lack of intimacy in your life? Are you in a financial bind and, at least while you are eating, do you think you can ignore the pile of bills you cannot pay?

Are you in a job which offers no challenge or purpose to your life? Is your job overly demanding and you feel overwhelmed? Are you home with toddlers and constantly having to fix bottles, snacks, meals, pick up toys, and deal with demanding children?

If you turn to food to handle these situations, then you are weighing your emotions. If you are able to handle your emotions unrelated to food, the outcome is probably more positive. Take time to reflect on your life. How can you get off the emotional roller coaster on which you find yourself? If a situation cannot be changed, how can you deal with the emotion other than turning to food? Write down your thoughts, set a goal, and then work to accomplish the goal.

If you are physically able, substitute activity for those times when you find yourself reaching for food in response to your emotions. You can walk, ride a bike, swim, or work out with a low impact aerobics video. If you have physical and/or health limitations, reach for a craft project, listen to a favorite tape, or read a book to get your mind off of food.

What are you weighing today besides pounds and ounces? Perhaps it is a bad day at work; someone hurt your feelings; an event brought to mind a painful memory. Maybe you would like to have a successful career that challenges you; instead, you are working at a job where you are not happy. Maybe you are a career person and wish you could be home with your family or retire early or perhaps travel. Maybe you are having financial problems and each week is a struggle. Maybe you struggle with loneliness. Maybe you struggle with your health.

You have quite a load to carry, but I have some good news for you! In Hebrews 12:1-2 the Bible says, "Let us throw off everything [not one thing, not two things, but *everything*] that hinders and . . . so easily entangles, and let us run with perseverance the race marked out for us. Let us fix our eyes on Jesus, the Author and Perfecter of our faith."

Use the lines at the end of this chapter to write down what positive steps you plan to take to overcome or change these problems or emotions which weigh you down. What will *you* do to "throw off everything that hinders"?

Friends, the race is marked. With the *Weigh to Win Weight Management System,* we know the route to take. We may stumble and fall, but if we will have perseverance we can finish the race. Some of us cannot even see the finish line yet; we have to run the race one mile marker at a time.

Get some exercise, think positive thoughts, and have a great day!

****

Yes, I will work to "throw off everything that hinders" by taking the following positive steps:

1. _____

2. _____

3. _____

4. _____

TEN

Heading Off Binges at the Pass

Binge eating poses the same threat to your weight loss efforts as a typhoon does to island dwellers and a tornado to people on the plains: it threatens to destroy a lifetime of effort. But binges, unlike forces of nature, are controllable, psychologically motivated events. Even though you do not prevent the binge from beginning, you can take precautions to lessen its damage.

People react differently to binges. Some people regard an extra serving of fruit as a binge; others do not feel that they have binged unless they have eaten uncontrollably for hours or even days.

Binge eating usually begins with a combination of moods such as boredom and anger. Binges start small, build up quickly, and are more likely to occur when you skip meals. Negative moods and skipped meals set the stage for binge eating.

Binge eating almost always takes place at home. It sometimes occurs after you return home from having just eaten a good, nutritious meal in a restaurant. If your attitude about the meal is negative, the *martyr syndrome* sets in. You feel deprived because the others with you raved over their fattening desserts while you refused one and ate broiled chicken breast, baked potato, and a salad. So, you went home and "rewarded" yourself with the chocolate cake from Susie's sixteenth birthday party.

Binge eating usually occurs at night. Do you find evenings the most difficult time of the day to control your eating? You are often weary by that time, weaker physically and emotionally from the day's events, and Satan hides in the shroud of darkness to try to defeat you. Ephesians 5:11 warns, "Have nothing to do with the fruitless deeds of darkness, but rather expose them." If you give in to nighttime binge eating, the binge will probably extend far into the next day.

Binge eating is almost always hidden from others. You would be embarrassed if others saw how much you were eating, and so you may go to great lengths to hide your actions. Binges often begin with small or moderate amounts of a food you particularly enjoy, but then go on to include larger amounts of almost anything.

During a binge, you rarely can account for how much you are eating, either during or afterward. You block out the information because you are not ready emotionally to handle the fact that you have just eaten a dozen cookies and are headed for more.

With this in mind, *Weigh to Win* has developed a five-step Binge Control Program:

☐ Step 1: *Distraction*. When you feel the need for food which would put you over the amount of food your body needs for the day, or when the food is not on the *Weigh to Win* Rainbow Food Plan, try distraction first by turning to something other than food.

Distraction can help to break your preoccupation with eating. Create distraction by changing your activity and your environment. If you are in the kitchen when the urge to eat strikes, go to the basement, the bedroom, or the backyard—go any place where you will not be in contact with food. If you are watching television when the urge to eat strikes, turn it off and put on your favorite music. If you are reading, try television. If you are cleaning, turn to a hobby.

Keep your Bible handy. I hope that you have a well-read Bible in which you have highlighted positive verses which give you strength. Just flip through and read those verses. Tell the Lord that you realize He is not going to keep you from heading for the kitchen if you choose to do so. Tell Him that you do not want to give in and be out of control with your eating, and that you need for Him to give you strength right now to get you through this moment. Pray away your urge to overeat.

Do anything which will change your environment and occupy your mind. In changing both environment and activity, you take into account the fact that your urge to eat is a response to your present situation. By changing the situation, you can limit your urge to eat.

☐ Step 2: *Delay.* Set a timer and wait at least ten minutes after you experience the urge to eat. The ten-minute wait will provide time to think; it can help to break the hold your preoccupation with food has on you and give you the opportunity to become interested in other things. Waiting ten minutes can also prove to you that you are still in control. When the bell rings, if you feel more time is needed to get the urge to eat under control, set the timer for another ten minutes.

I sometimes talk to myself out loud. "Okay, Lynn, you have made it through ten minutes and, if you can make it through one ten-minute segment, you can make it through another." I seldom have to set the timer a third time, but everyone is different. If you need to set it several times, do it!

☐ Step 3: *Detour*. If you do eat, choose a food which is *not* on your "favorite food" list. Choosing a *nonpreferred* food is a very important part of this anti-binge program. Because your resistance is low when you are set to binge, you may experience a tendency to eat far too much of your favorite foods. If you do, you are, in effect, rewarding yourself for allowing your eating to get out of control.

Take a few moments to complete the following chart. Make a list in column 1 of the foods which you particularly enjoy. You would find these foods easy to turn to when you are in danger of bingeing. In column 2, make a list of nonpreferred foods. *Do not* list foods which you cannot tolerate at all. *Do* list foods which you enjoy, but do not reach for when feeling the desire to binge.

<table>
<tr><th>Column 1
Dangerous Binge Foods</th><th>Column 2
Less Preferred Foods</th></tr>
<tr><td>_____</td><td>_____</td></tr>
<tr><td>_____</td><td>_____</td></tr>
<tr><td>_____</td><td>_____</td></tr>
<tr><td>_____</td><td>_____</td></tr>
<tr><td>_____</td><td>_____</td></tr>
</table>

Do not look at this as a "Look what I have to give up for this carrot stick" exercise. Instead, pat yourself on the back each time you choose a food from your less preferred list, instead of one from your binge list. You can feel good that you made a nutritious choice. Thank the Lord for helping you.

☐ Step 4: *Downsizing.* If you are fighting a binge and weaken, take just a small amount of the food which you are eating. If you go back for more, again take the smallest possible helping. The message in this is:

DO ALL YOU CAN TO MAKE CERTAIN
THAT EVERY TIME YOU EAT
YOU HAVE GIVEN YOURSELF AN OPPORTUNITY
TO DRAW THE FINAL LINE.

I know that I can very easily binge on half a loaf of raisin bread. When this urge comes, if I have not been able to fully get it under control, I have learned to just take out one slice. Then, I close the loaf, put the twist tie back on the wrapper, and place the bread in the back of the freezer. If I start to go for another slice, I have to get it out of the cold freezer and undo the twist tie. Every added deterrent gives me seconds to gain control over what I am doing. In times past, I would take the loaf to the table, leave it open, and eat slice after slice, usually loaded with butter or cream cheese. When I was finished, I could not even tell you how much I had eaten.

This downsizing technique helps to keep my eating controllable. If I do binge, it is not going to be a very big one. Remember that *Weigh to Win* teaches you behaviors which will help you not only get trim but stay trim, and this is one of those behaviors which needs to be practiced.

☐ Step 5: *Deliberateness.* Consider anything which you have eaten to be water over the dam. Do not dwell on it. Get out your *Weigh to Win* Rainbow Food Plan book and plan out your very next meal. Make it especially luscious with some of your favorite *Weigh to Win* recipes.

Give Yourself Positive Messages

If you have started to snack and realize that you are deviating from your eating plan, it is important that you give yourself positive messages. What types of statements could you say to yourself to keep from feeling hopelessly defeated? You might recognize that you ate only one piece of cake instead of the two or three you would have eaten in the past. Admit that you made a mistake, but tell yourself that continuing the binge will not make it better. Resolve to sit down immediately and plan your next healthy meal. Tell yourself that you are not going to let this minor setback cause you to give up on all that you have accomplished.

Many binge eaters tell themselves that they have done "a terrible thing" and have proven that they have "no willpower." These are self-indulgent statements which merely set them up for more binge eating. God is not going to condemn anyone for eating a few extra slices of bread!

As a challenge, consider learning to control the responses which trigger your binge eating. Ask yourself, "How can I keep my eating within bounds?" Instead of making self-destructive statements, direct your thoughts to positive statements which help to keep your actions in check.

Summary

In summary, there are four basic principles to conquering binge eating.

☐ First, you must take steps to control your moods and plan your meals wisely.

☐ Second, you must prepare a strategy which will allow you to gain control of the urge to eat, so that you have the greatest possible number of opportunities to keep your eating within reasonable bounds. If you panic, you will be less likely to gain the control you need.

☐ Third, you must preplan and realize that bingeing means only that the first set of limits did not work. So, a second line of defense is needed to help control the panic and contain the damage done by binges.

☐ Finally, when bingeing slows down your weight control efforts, take the binge in stride and work to get back to healthy eating at the earliest possible moment. Do not give up!

**BINGEING DOES NOT CREATE DISASTER.
OVERREACTION TO BINGES IS THE MAJOR VILLAIN.**

Philippians 3:20 tells us, "We eagerly await a Savior . . . the Lord Jesus Christ, who, by the power that enables Him to bring everything under His control, will transform our lowly bodies so that they will be like His glorious body."

I look forward to the day when I no longer have the earthly struggle of continually working to overcome lifelong eating habits. Although God will not stop me from bingeing if I choose to do so, I am thankful that He is there to encourage and to help me to make good choices if I but ask.

The road is not always an easy one, but it is joy-filled as we gain confidence in our healthy new lifestyle. You, God, and *Weigh to Win* working together spell s-u-c-c-e-s-s.

ELEVEN

Taking the "Less" Out of "Hopeless"

"And we know that in all things God works for the good of those who love Him, who have been called according to His purpose" (Romans 8:28). All things? Even medical problems, even stress, even financial problems, even being overweight? Although our efforts to succeed sometimes seem hopeless, in this chapter we will be sharing some steps which are meant to help you take the "less" out of "hopeless."

Break New Ground with God

"Be still, and know that I am God," the psalmist writes in Psalm 46:10. Sometimes you can feel all alone in your weight loss effort, but you do have available a source of strength from your Heavenly Father. Try to remind yourself of the nearness of God. Breathe *in* His presence and breathe *out* your doubts. Quit trying to do everything on your own. Your willpower goes only so far. You can rely on the Lord to give you strength when you are weak. Breathe out the doubts which say, "I am probably going to fail anyway," and breathe *in* thoughts which say, "I can do everything through Him who gives me strength" (Philippians 4:13).

Restore Your Spirit from God's Word

Set aside time for Bible study. Revelation 3:8 says, "See, I have placed before you an open door that no one can shut." God's Word is like an open door and, if you will walk through it, you can gain wisdom, understanding, and guidance when you have difficult choices to make. Use a Bible concordance to look up Scripture references on self-control and discipline. Then spend time memorizing the verses most meaningful to you. Memorized Scripture is a powerful tool to use against Satan when he tries to defeat you. My favorite Scripture passage is Jeremiah 29:11-14:

> "For I know the plans I have for you," declares the Lord, "plans to prosper you and not to harm you, plans to give you hope and a future. Then you will call upon Me and come and pray to Me, and I will listen to you. You will seek Me and find Me when you seek Me with all your heart. I will be found by you," declares the Lord.

These verses give assurance that God wants the best for me and that He has a plan. He promises to be with me if I will seek Him with all my heart. This Scripture is packed with hope!

Remove Negative Ideas

Remove negative words from your vocabulary. Remember that the word *can't* usually means *won't*. Become aware of the times when you use "no" or "not" words such as *shouldn't, wouldn't, couldn't, didn't, don't,* or *never.* Try to think how you could rephrase negative statements with positive words. Instead of mournfully eyeing the brownie in the lunch line and crying, "I can't eat that," turn your thoughts around and say, "I could have that brownie, but I choose a healthy body instead!" Do you hear the difference?

I challenge you to keep a tally of how many times in an average day you use "no" words when you speak or write. You may be surprised at the negative thoughts which are unconsciously perforating your thinking. Positive thinking is learned just as negative thinking is. Which do you choose?

My husband's late grandmother was a dear Christian woman. Until cancer kept her mind and body from functioning normally, almost daily she visited shut-ins and anyone needing help or encouragement. I will never forget her saying one day that she had to make a conscious decision as she aged to not grow old *bitter* but to grow old *better*. After her husband was killed in a car accident when he was only in his forties, it would have been easy to become bitter with life. Instead, she chose the better way. As she helped others, she helped herself. We can choose to be *bitter* because we have to struggle with a weight problem; or we can choose to be *better* by taking control of negative thoughts and turning them around to achieve our weight loss goal.

Be Willing to Dream

Visualize yourself ten pounds thinner. Think about something which you have always wanted to do that is not food related, and take beginning steps to achieve it. Everyone has a talent or skill which needs to be used and developed. A poster in my office says:

> TO ACCOMPLISH GREAT THINGS,
> WE MUST NOT ONLY ACT BUT ALSO DREAM,
> NOT ONLY PLAN BUT ALSO BELIEVE.

Being willing to dream is risky. Perhaps you have had other dreams which did not turn out as you expected, and you may be afraid to dream again. If you do not dream about how good it will feel to be thinner, you will not achieve your weight loss goal. Do not be so afraid of failure that you sabotage your own success.

Is there something you have always wanted to do, but have been afraid to take the steps to accomplish? What about that art class you have always wanted to take? How about going back to school, taking golfing lessons, getting your pilot's license, or learning to ski? Take one step today to work toward accomplishing your dream. Make a phone call, set up an appointment, review your budget to see how the cost of lessons could be worked in. Ultimately, we do what we want to do. If you want something enough, you will find a way to accomplish it.

Learn to Be Patient

You did not become overweight overnight—even though it may seem as if you just woke up one morning and all that fat was there. A long journey is easier to travel if you build on each week's success. Add up the total pounds you have lost and then rejoice in your success. Set small goals for yourself. Inch by inch, it is a cinch. Before you know it you will be thin and healthy.

Psalm 37:7 says, "Be still before the Lord and wait patiently for Him." In the past, your impatience has led you to try fad diets which promised a fast weight loss. You now know that the only way to lose weight safely and permanently is with a program such as the *Weigh to Win* Rainbow Food Plan which allows you to lose weight gradually through a well-balanced way of eating which can be followed throughout your lifetime. Make fitness a focus of your life.

At the support group I was attending throughout my weight loss, one woman said she had lost fifty-five pounds. I thought to myself, "If she can do it, so can I." Her success gave me hope. I want my weight loss—120 pounds after a twenty-year battle with weight—to give you hope that no matter how many times you have tried in the past, you can and will succeed this time.

Twelve

How Your Thoughts Control Your Actions

You are behind in your work. The tension builds as you begin to realize that you will never be able to catch up. Negative thoughts creep in and you begin to feel like a failure. The day is ruined and so you head for the coffee pot. Since everything else is going wrong, you might as well have some toast with the coffee. You fill both slots on the toaster with bread and then reach for the margarine and jelly in the refrigerator. The toast pops up and you put in two more slices. Suddenly realizing that you have just eaten four slices of bread at one sitting, you think this proves you are a failure. You feel worse than you did before you headed for the coffee pot; your self-esteem takes a plunge; and you eat even more.

Thoughts ◊ Feelings ◊ Actions ◊ Reactions

This chain reaction is universal. You are not the only one who eats uncontrollably at times. Thoughts lead to feelings, feelings to actions, and actions to reactions. In this case, a negative thought triggered a negative feeling which led to negative actions and reactions.

If only you had thought, "Even though I am not going to be able to finish my work, at least I have made a good beginning," you might have felt better about yourself and continued to work instead of turning to food.

Thoughts ◊ Feelings ◊ Actions ◊ Reactions are all links in the chain of learned eating behaviors. If you can be successful in changing even one link in the chain, the end result will be a step toward overcoming the eating habits which keep you overweight.

Most people who habitually overeat make mistakes in the way they think about food. Becoming aware of these mistakes will help you break the chain of eating responses which lead to problem eating.

Incorrect Information

The first mistake is incorrect information. There is as much myth as truth in popular ideas about food and weight loss. For instance, many people believe that they have to be hungry to lose weight, that toasting bread reduces its calories, that food eaten after 6 o'clock in the evening is more fattening than food eaten earlier in the day, that washing pasta removes all of its starch, and that bread is bad for you if you are trying to lose weight. The facts are much different.

If you are hungry, you are much more likely to overeat. To effectively lose weight, you must eat enough food to meet your nutritional needs and also control your physical hunger. The *Weigh to Win* Rainbow Food Plan meets these requirements by providing you with the guidelines for nutritionally balanced meals and special unlimited foods to which you may turn if you still feel hungry. Toasting bread removes moisture, not calories. Food eaten after 6 o'clock in the evening has no more calories in it than the same food eaten earlier in the day. Food eaten in the evening becomes fattening only if it is eaten in excess of daily energy needs. Washing spaghetti may remove some vitamins but not much starch. If you are to succeed at losing weight, you need to work from facts, not fallacies.

Dichotomous Thinking

The second mistake is dichotomous thinking. Have you noticed that when your work is not completed you feel *all bad* and when the job is done you feel *all good?* You never feel a *little* bad or a *little* good. When you are *all bad,* you are beyond hope; when you are *all good,* you cannot err.

Do you consider every extra bite to be a clear sign that you are weak-willed and destined for failure? Does one nibble make you feel that all is lost and there is no way back from the smallest mistake? Have you fallen into the trap of thinking that since you overate at breakfast, the entire day was a loss? And that since you ruined the day, the week was "down the tubes"? Do you sometimes think that you will *never* change because you will *always* be just the same? For people who think this way, everything is black or white. You should try to think how much better off you will be if you are willing to give yourself credit for being human and then take small mistakes in stride.

To avoid the terrible trap of dichotomous thinking, which is a common trick Satan tries to use on us, you should consider a momentary poor choice of food as a temporary and minor detour on your weight loss journey, and then go on to plan better choices the rest of the day.

Negatives versus Positives

A third mistake is to emphasize negatives and disregard positives. You have been on the *Weigh to Win Weight Man-*

agement System program for three days and have eaten break-fast, lunch, and dinner exactly as planned. You even planned healthy snacks for between meals. But, after dinner, while visiting friends, you ate a piece of banana cream pie and it was not prepared *Weigh to Win* style. When you got home that night, you felt you had done it again—fallen off the wagon before the journey had barely begun. To console yourself, you ate a dozen chocolate chip cookies (or another favorite binge food) which you had bought "for the kids" and washed them down with a large glass of milk. You were already quite full from dinner, but you ate anyway.

You might have told yourself that you just made a mistake which points to an overeating habit not yet under control, and that you were going to have to be more careful in the future. You might have consoled yourself by thinking how well you had done all day long. You might even have given yourself credit for having just eaten one piece of pie—not two or three! Instead, you magnified the negatives and forgot about the positives.

Learn to keep your mistakes in perspective.

Terminal Thinking

A fourth mistake is terminal thinking. When you came home after the pie-eating incident, did you wonder *why* you had made such a mistake? Did you berate yourself for being weak and having no willpower? Did you tell yourself that you were just born to be fat because you had no self-control? This kind of terminal thinking keeps you from making rational decisions. Instead of thinking about *why* you got into the situation, you could have analyzed *how* you could have handled yourself differently. *Why* questions do little more than point blame and verify failure. *How* questions start the problem-solving process.

Reversed Thinking

The fifth mistake is reversed thinking. You would like to work on your weight problem, but you have struggled with depression for the past several months. You tell yourself, "When I feel better about myself, then I will start to do something for me." This is a classic example of reversed thinking. You believe that your mood must change *before* you change your behavior; however, your moods are more likely a *result* of your actions. Each time you make a poor food choice, you add to your feeling of depression.

You put the proverbial cart before the horse saying, "I will get serious about my weight loss when my spouse and I have a better relationship," or "when the kids go back to school," or "when the pressure is off at work." This is like trying to complete the roof of a building without having built the walls; there is no chance for success.

To unscramble reversed thoughts, it is necessary to think of first things first, of cause and effect. To *feel* better, you must change what you *do*. To change what you *do,* you must change the way you *think*. We are reminded in Romans 12:2, "Do not conform any longer to the pattern of this world, but be transformed by the renewing of your mind."

To lose weight, you must change what you *eat*. To change your use of food, you must learn to control the *habits* which trigger your desire to eat. Reversed thinking backs you into a box with no way out; straight thinking is the only way for you to successfully reach your goal.

Fatalistic Thinking

The sixth and possibly the worst mistake is fatalism. Have you ever heard of self-fulfilling prophecies? Sometimes we have ourselves so convinced that we are going to fail that we actually do things which lead to inevitable failure.

Use the following written exercise to reveal how much fatalism has crept into your thinking. After each statement circle a number 1 if you would say, "Yes, that's me! That is what I think." Circle a number 2 if you would say, "No, that isn't me at all."

That's me That's not
         me

1	2	1. I learned my eating behaviors as a child, and you can't teach an old dog new tricks.
1	2	2. If I think that someone does not like or respect me, I think there is something wrong with me.
1	2	3. It is normal to turn to food as a response to all emotions.
1	2	4. It is always my fault when things do not turn out as I expected.
1	2	5. Things just happen to me; I can't do anything to improve situations.
1	2	6. I do not expect to be successful at changing my eating habits and losing weight.
1	2	7. I cannot control my eating when I am upset.
1	2	8. I am always the one who misses out when good things happen.

If you put a number 1 for even one of these statements, you may be creating unnecessary problems for yourself. Clear these thoughts right out of your mind. When you start thinking this way, talk to yourself to set your thinking straight.

Pretend you are a member of a debate team. The other team has just made a case for your negative thought and your job is to prove them wrong. Weaken the strength of the negative thought by refuting it in your own words and then develop positive, alternative messages. If you confidently expect positive results, you will act in a positive way.

Straight Thinking

Positive thoughts must lead to positive action. "Day by day, I am getting better and better" is a statement which, though positive, does not lead to action. Instead, use phrases which suggest constructive action. For example, negative thinking would say, "The women in the Ladies' Missionary Circle are so creative. I'm not very good at making crafts, so I just won't go." Positive action thinking would say, "Different people have different talents. I will find something to contribute to the group, and I will learn from others who have abilities which I lack."

Negative thinking would say, "I cannot control my eating at parties. I always make a pig of myself. Everyone has to be thinking, 'Look at that fat guy with his plate loaded with food.' I just won't go to the party so I don't embarrass myself." Positive action thinking would say, "If I have a healthy snack at home I will not be as likely to overeat at the party. Instead of focusing on the food, I am going to have fun with my friends. I will go late and leave early."

To keep the mistakes mentioned in this chapter from hindering your weight loss success, you need to make effective plans that start with facts, not fallacies. Think in terms of partial success, not of total victory or total defeat. Develop a balanced view of yourself, giving your assets their full credit while admitting your weaknesses.

Plan how to take advantage of the opportunities posed by

challenges rather than asking why situations make you feel powerless. If you are feeling powerless, remember, "When we were still powerless, Christ died for [us]" (Romans 5:6). And, "The voice of the Lord is powerful. . . . The Lord gives strength to His people" (Psalm 29:4, 11). Plan a course of action rather than expecting results before action.

Straight thinking involves knowing exactly where you are beginning, what you hope to accomplish, and the steps you can take to move from where you are to where you want to be. Your goal must be specific. The knowledge of where you are must be precise. And the steps you take must be small, positive, and all in the right direction. According to Proverbs 14:15, "A prudent man gives thought to his steps." Ask the Lord to help you with your thought life so that your thoughts will lead to positive action instead of negative action.

Thirteen

Label Reading Made Easy

The sign proclaims that the french fries contain no cholesterol. The peanut butter jar reads "No cholesterol." The blue label on a bunch of bananas also says "No cholesterol." The soup mix package claims that it is "Lite." The pancake mix box says "Light." The health food cookies package claims they are "Sugar-free." The turkey sausage claims to be "Eighty-five percent fat-free." The fast food hamburger touts that it is "Ninety-one percent fat-free." The meat package in the grocery store says "Extra lean."

What do these terms mean? Can we believe the claims? In a list of ingredients, what does "partially hydrogenated vegetable oil" mean? Unless you are armed with a basic knowledge of reading food labels, you are a sitting duck for the marketing ploys of food distributors.

If you are going to lose weight successfully and maintain your weight loss for the rest of your life, you must learn to read nutrition information on food labels and not depend on marketing slogans. To do this, you need factual information from reputable sources. If you choose to dig a little deeper than the information contained in this chapter, the Food and Drug Administration has a great number of helpful articles, many free of charge, available through the Superintendent of Documents, Government Printing Office, Washington, D.C. 20402. The American Dietetic Association, 216 W. Jackson Street, Suite 800, Chicago, Illinois 60606, and your local Dairy Council are also very good sources of accurate nutrition information.

A Hands-on Approach to Food Labels

The purpose of this chapter is to give you a hands-on approach to reading food labels. I don't wish to delve into the food additives and preservatives controversy; it is my personal opinion that most food additives are safe when consumed in moderation and are certainly a better alternative than allowing the bacteria to grow which causes food poisoning. I realize this may offend some health purists, but I tend to take a more middle-of-the-road approach to this controversial subject.

Actually, I would enjoy growing all of the foods needed to feed my family, raising our own meat, and milking our own cows, and then processing the food under strict sanitary conditions with no preservatives or food additives. The reality of work schedules, and the lack of equipment, lands, buildings, and livestock necessary to accomplish such a task, leaves me no alternative but to make the best choices available from my local grocery store. Buying expensive organically grown foods just does not fit into our food budget; also, I have found little documented medical proof that there is any substantial nutritional advantage to choosing such foods.

Because nutrition education is a major thrust of *Weigh to Win,* this chapter is critical to your weight loss success. You will find it helpful to check the labels on some foods in your pantry or freezer. You may find foods that do not have an ingredient label. The general rule of *Weigh to Win* is, if there is no label, do not eat it. Food labeling laws may be changing in the near future but, as of this writing, the law provides *standards of identity* which excuses the manufacturers from listing ingredients for some items. Standards of identity exist for common foods which at one time were often prepared at home. The basic recipe was understood by almost everyone for such items as bread and mayonnaise. Now, however, few people make these foods at home and commercial recipes may be far different than what was included in the original recipe. Labels on foods considered *standards of identity* are done voluntarily by the manufacturer.

Know Your Terminology

When reading food labels, look for the word *imitation*. Current law requires that foods which are a substitute for, but nutritionally inferior to the original, be labeled imitation. If you eat imitation cheese instead of real cheese, you will not be getting the same nutrients. Imitation foods are not necessarily lower in calories.

Watch for products labeled *natural, organic,* or *health foods*. The federal government has no legal definition for these terms. Manufacturers use the terms indiscriminately, often to justify charging you a higher price.

The term *light* or *lite* has no legal definition. The "light" pancake mix you bought may just be lighter in texture than another brand. "Light" olive oil may only be lighter in color with no reduction in calories. "Lite" soups may be only slightly lower in sodium, with no difference in calories. Whenever I see the word *lite* or *light* I ask myself, "Lighter than what?" If the lite ice cream still has 200 calories per serving and a 55 percent fat content, then it is not a dietetic product, even if it does contain fewer calories than the original product.

Cholesterol Confusion

Then there is the confusing cholesterol issue. Everything seems to be labeled "No cholesterol." If the product contains no cholesterol, does that mean it is safe to eat in any amount? Does the cholesterol in your blood come from the cholesterol you eat? The fact is that most of the cholesterol in your blood is manufactured by your own body. Your body produces approximately 600–1,500 milligrams of cholesterol per day from the fats, protein, and carbohydrates you eat. You also ingest cholesterol by eating foods which contain cholesterol. Both the cholesterol you eat and the cholesterol your own body produces end up in your bloodstream.

Cholesterol is found in all animals because it is necessary for the formation of cell membranes and other vital substances. Thus, all animal products—meat, eggs, poultry, fish, and dairy products—contain cholesterol. No plant-derived food contains cholesterol. Therefore, peanut butter, bananas, and vegetable oil cannot contain cholesterol. Labeling them as a "No cholesterol" food is just a marketing tactic playing on the new awareness of the cholesterol issue.

Although our bodies produce cholesterol from the fats, protein, and carbohydrates we eat, the biggest culprit in our diet is fat. The more fat we eat, whether the food contains grams of cholesterol or not, the greater chance we will have of increasing the cholesterol our own body produces.

A label may accurately say "No cholesterol" and still be a high fat food which contributes to an elevated cholesterol level in some individuals. A bottle of "No cholesterol" vegetable oil is certainly a better choice than lard or shortening, but it is still pure fat and provides just as many calories. Those french fries cooked in "No cholesterol" oil offer no magic formula that eating them, or any other similarly prepared food in excess of your body's nutritional needs, will not elevate your cholesterol level—especially if a low fat diet is not being followed on a daily basis. Nor are they lower in calories than french fries prepared with saturated fats.

Fat Facts

Although we need to be aware of high cholesterol foods, our emphasis should be more on the consumption of fat. Only about 33 percent of the average adult daily caloric intake should be from fat. When reading food labels, look for the following terms: lard, butter, margarine, coconut oil, cocoa butter, palm kernel oil, beef tallow, palm oil, vegetable oil, cottonseed oil, olive oil, peanut oil, canola oil, or vegetable shortening. If the term *hydrogenated* or *partially hydrogenated* is used, it means the manufacturer has used a chemical to harden the liquid oil and therefore increase saturation. In the past, this process of increasing saturation was thought to increase the risk of heart disease, but current research shows that it may not increase this risk when eaten in appropriate amounts.

We need fat in our diet because it carries with it certain nutrients; it also lubricates the skin and digestive tract. However, the average adult consumes far too much fat on a daily basis.

Sugar-Free?

"Sugarless" or "Sugar-free" claims on packaging simply mean the food has no added sucrose or white table sugar. The term does not mean that the product is lower in calories or that other sweeteners such as corn syrup, honey, brown sugar, molasses, invert sugar, sorghum, mannitol, or sorbitol have not been used. A package claiming a "good-for-you" cookie which contained "no sugar" showed "pure, unrefined cane juice" in the list of ingredients. No sugar? Often fruit juice concentrates are used to sweeten products. Fruit juices contain fructose, a natural sugar. In concentrated form, these "natural sugars" can pack a lot of calories into a product. Honey is metabolized by the body the same as sugar and even contains slightly more calories. Check the list of ingredients for words ending in *-ose* such as *sucrose, dextrose, lactose, maltose, glucose,* and *fructose.* All are forms of sugar. The sign at some frozen yogurt stores proclaims "100 percent Nutrasweet," but a list of ingredients, if you can get one, often shows other sweeteners.

Studying Food Labels

Now, let's get down to the "nuts and bolts" of label reading. Gather from your pantry and freezer food items which have nutritional information on the labels and answer the following questions:

1. How many servings are in the container? What is the serving size? How many calories are there per serving?
Jackie was new to the *Weigh to Win Weight Management System* and a novice at label reading. She thought she had made a good choice when she purchased a can of "lite" cherry pie filling. The label read "fifty calories per serving." Jackie neglected to read on and learn that there were eight servings in the can. She had eaten the entire can, consuming 400 calories instead of 50.

Calories are always listed *per serving* and product labels frequently indicate that there is more than one serving. For example, carbonated diet soft drinks containing 10 percent fruit juice are usually put in a twelve-ounce can. The label on the can indicates that there are fifteen calories per serving. A closer look reveals that the manufacturer considers there to be two servings per can. Therefore, if you drink the whole can, you have consumed thirty calories.

I recently fell victim to this marketing trap myself. Many single-serving-type dietetic yogurts show the amount of calories on the front of the container. I found a sugar-free and nonfat yogurt in an eight-ounce container which read "only fifty calories" in large lettering on the front of the package. In very small print, which I had overlooked, were two important words— "per serving." Thinking that it was grand to be able to eat eight ounces of yogurt for only fifty calories, I took a few home to try. It has become a habit to study a label on a new food before I eat it, so I automatically turned to the back of the container. There I discovered that there were fifty calories in a *four-ounce* serving with *two servings* per container.

2. How many grams of carbohydrates are listed? Are the grams broken down into simple and complex carbohydrates?

Simple carbohydrates are sugars. If the food product contains a large percentage of simple carbohydrates, you need to realize that you are consuming sugar, even though the product may claim to be sugar-free. Approximately four grams of sugar equal one teaspoon; twelve grams equal one tablespoon. Carefully check your cereal box labels. The best choices are cereals with no more than five grams of sucrose per serving.

3. How many grams of fat are listed? What percentage of the calories in the product come from fat?

The mathematical formula for figuring the percentage of calories from fat is really quite simple. There are nine calories in one gram of fat. A label may indicate that there are only three grams of fat per serving. This seems like a very small amount. However, multiply nine calories times the three grams of fat and discover a total of twenty-seven calories. If the product contains only forty total calories per serving, three grams of fat would mean that 68 percent of the total amount of calories in the serving comes from fat calories. This would not be a low-fat product. If the product contained ninety calories per serving with three grams of fat, only 30 percent of the calories in the product would come from fat, making it a lower fat product. You need to look at every label of every food you eat to determine fat content.

The food label of a package of turkey sausage claimed the product was 85 percent fat-free, but there were three grams of fat in a fifty-calorie serving, making the percentage of calories from fat 54 percent. The label indicated that three types of fat were added to the product. What the manufacturer of the product meant was that the package contained 15 percent added fat *by weight*. Percentage of fat by weight and percentage of calories from fat give two very different perspectives. Turkey is one of the lower fat meats to choose, but it still contains fat. When you add 15 percent more fat (by weight) to it, you get the 54 percent calories from fat which told the whole story.

Does this mean you should never eat a food with over 30 percent of its calories coming from fat? No, but it does mean that no more than 30 percent of the total calories you consume in a day should come from fat. If you eat a one-ounce slice of Swiss cheese, you are eating a product which is approximately 80 percent fat. This does not mean that you can never have a slice of cheese. It does mean that if you do have that slice of cheese, you had better choose other foods throughout the day which are very low in fat, or you will go over the amount of fat you should eat in a day.

Fortunately, if you are following the *Weigh to Win* Rainbow Food Plan, the amount of fat you eat is figured automatically and kept in balance by the choices allowed. Figuring the percentage of fat calories becomes more critical when choosing appropriate foods for lifetime maintenance or when determining if a food is truly a dietetic food which may be counted toward the Freedom to Choose calories allowed on the food plan.

4. How many milligrams of sodium are listed?

It is best to limit your sodium to 2,000-3,000 milligrams per day. With this in mind, ask yourself if this food is a good choice. Knowing that avoiding all sodium is virtually impossible, consuming one food which contains 1,500 grams of sodium per serving may not be a very wise choice.

If you do not have high blood pressure or a problem with water retention, sodium content may not be a major factor for you. However, it is always good to be aware of what is best for our health. One teaspoon of table salt contains approximately 2,000 milligrams of sodium.

Many prepackaged dinners which require no refrigeration contain very high amounts of sodium. The packaging entices a dieter with "under 300 calories" but then the nutrition information on the label indicates 1,800 milligrams of sodium.

5. What are the first three ingredients in the order given?

Sometimes you will find a nutritional breakdown of a food product, but no list of ingredients given. If the manufacturer is not willing to list what is in the product, do not eat it.

Ingredients are listed in order by *weight*. The product contains more of the first ingredient listed than the second ingredient, more of the second ingredient than the third ingredient, and so on. If the first or second ingredient listed is sugar or a form of sugar as previously listed in this chapter, it certainly cannot be considered a dietetic food, no matter what the packaging indicates.

This list of ingredients is very important in making wise

food choices. The food label of an extra lean hamburger a fast food restaurant began marketing indicated that the second ingredient was water. Adding water would certainly decrease the calories in the hamburger, but a three-ounce portion of this type of hamburger would not give the same nutrients as a three-ounce portion of a 100 percent beef hamburger. Further reading showed carrageenan added as a thickener, with beef flavoring as the fourth ingredient. If the hamburger was all beef, why does "beef flavoring" need to be added? You must always be on your guard.

The list of ingredients for a "fat-free" muffin indicated that sugar was the first ingredient. This would not be a dietetic product.

Avoid Fat and Sugar

Overweight people have what I call a "double whammy." We not only need to watch the fat in our diet, but we also need to limit the amount of sugar in all forms. Sugar is calorically dense with little nutritional value. This does not mean that we can never eat anything sweet tasting; it just means that we must make choices. Many recipes can be made with artificial sweeteners or using fruit such as apples and bananas in allowed portions to make a delightfully sweet dessert. Do not be taken in by foods claiming to be "fat free." They may still be very high in sugar and calories.

I find label reading fascinating. The more I learn, the more I realize I need to learn. I read and study to keep my knowledge up to date. I look at all packaging claims with skepticism until I can see that the claims are factual. You need to take responsibility for your own health by learning to read and understand nutrition information and then pray as the psalmist in Psalm 119:66, "Teach me knowledge and good judgment."

FOURTEEN

Determining Your Basal Metabolic Rate

I frequently hear people complain that they are not able to lose weight because of a "slow metabolism." *Weigh to Win* stresses how important it is for you to eat *all* the food coming to you on the Rainbow Food Plan, and that the food portions are *mandatory* to give your body what it needs nutritionally in order to avoid a slowed metabolism. But what is this thing called "metabolism"?

I can almost imagine my "metabolism" being a little black box with a needle gauge on it somewhere inside my body, measuring how much I eat and how much I exercise. It then indicates on the gauge if my "metabolism" is slow, normal, or fast. After this analysis takes place, fat cells are either spewed out or sucked up to cause me to gain or lose weight.

No, metabolism is not a little black box, but it can still seem rather mystical, unless we take time to try to understand what happens inside our bodies on a daily basis.

Is Your Energy Budget Unbalanced?

If you consume 3,500 calories *more* than your body uses in energy, you will *gain* approximately one pound of fat. Conversely, if you consume 3,500 calories *fewer* than your body requires for energy over a period of days or weeks, you will *lose* approximately one pound of fat. The way a person becomes overweight is by having an unbalanced energy budget—that is, by eating more food energy than is spent on metabolic and muscle activities.

You can easily figure your energy *intake* if you are following the *Weigh to Win Weight Management System,* because the Rainbow Food Plan is approximately 1,200 calories per day for a woman and 1,700 calories per day for a man. If you were not on a reduced calorie program, would you know how many calories you should eat to maintain your weight? Do you know how many calories you would have to be eating right now just to maintain your existing weight?

The United States Committee on Recommended Daily Allowances [RDA] and the Canadian Ministry of Health and Welfare have published recommended energy intakes for various age and sex groups. However, the range of energy needs is so broad that it is impossible even to guess an individual's needs without knowing something about the person's lifestyle. Taller people, on an average, need more energy intake; shorter people, less. Older people generally need less due to both slowed metabolism and reduced activity, with the number of calories diminishing by about 5 percent per decade beyond age thirty. It is impossible to determine any person's energy need within such a wide range without studying each individual.

The Components of Energy Output

In this chapter we will be concentrating on the two components of energy output: basal metabolic rate and voluntary muscle activities. You will need a calculator, pencil, and paper in order to figure your individual energy output.

You can get an estimate of your energy budget by monitoring your food intake over a minimum of a week's time and then adding together the two components of energy output. Compare intake versus output to determine the approximate state of your energy budget. If your intake is less than your output, you should lose weight. If your output is less than your intake, you should gain weight. If your intake and output are balanced, you should maintain your weight.

Estimating Your Basal Metabolic Rate

What is metabolism and how does it affect each one of us? The correct term is BMR or "basal metabolic rate." Basal metabolism is "the sum total of all the cellular activities that are necessary to sustain life, including respiration, circulation, and new tissue formation, and excluding digestion and voluntary activities."[1] Basal metabolism is the largest component of the average person's daily energy expenditure. The basal metabolic rate supports the work which goes on all the time in the body, without conscious awareness: the beating of the heart, the inhaling and exhaling of air, the maintenance of body temperature, and the sending of nerve and hormonal messages to direct these activities. These are the basal processes which maintain life. A person whose total energy needs are 2,000 calories a day spends as many as 1,200-1,400 of these calories to support basal metabolism.

First, to estimate your BMR or basal metabolic rate, you will need to know your weight in kilograms. One kilogram is about 2.2 pounds. So, take your current weight and divide it by 2.2 to figure the equivalent of your weight in kilograms. As an example, John is down to his goal weight and is a slim, healthy, 150 pounds. John takes his 150-pound weight and divides it by 2.2 pounds per kilogram to get his weight in kilograms which would be 68.

Second, multiply your weight in kilograms by 1.0 if you are a man or .9 if you are a woman. This formula is called the BMR factor. This number gives you the approximate number of calories spent *per hour* for your basal metabolism. Taking our previous example, John multiples his 68 kilograms of weight times the BMR factor of 1.0 for men to determine that his body uses 68 calories per hour for basal metabolism. If Alice also weighs 68 kilograms, she would multiply 68 times the BMR factor of .9 for women to arrive at an answer of 61 calories spent per hour for basal metabolism.

Third, multiply the calories used in one hour by the hours in a day. This figure gives you the approximate number of calories you use *each day* for basal metabolism. Example: John just determined that he uses 68 calories per hour. Sixty-eight calories per hour multiplied by twenty-four hours equals 1,632 calories *per day* spent for basal metabolism. Alice would take her 61 calories per hour times twenty-four hours to arrive at a figure of 1,464.

What was your answer? The number you determined for yourself represents the approximate number of calories your body spends each day just to sustain life through the basically unconscious activities of breathing, pumping your heart, and forming new tissue. For the most part, you are not even aware of your heart pumping or your lungs filling with air, although you would be aware if any of these functions suddenly stopped! Each day your body does a lot more than perform just these functions.

Estimating Calories Spent for Voluntary Muscle Activity

Your body also spends calories by *voluntary muscle activity*. To estimate the number of calories you as an individual spend on voluntary muscle activity, you will need to answer a few questions.

Your Occupation and Daily Activities

_____ 1. If you usually walk to and from work or shopping, at least one-half mile each way, give yourself 1 point.

_____ 2. If you usually take the stairs rather than use elevators or escalators, give yourself 1 point.

_____ 3. How would you best describe the type of physical activity involved in your job or daily household routine?

Choose only one of the following:

(a) If most of your workday is spent in office work, light physical activity, or housework, give yourself 0 points.

(b) If most of your workday is spent in farm activities, moderate physical activity, brisk walking, or comparable activities, give yourself 4 points.

(c) If your typical workday includes several hours of heavy physical activity such as shoveling or lifting, give yourself 9 points.

Your Leisure Activities

_____ 4. If you do several hours of gardening or lawn work each week, give yourself 1 point.

_____ 5. If you fish or hunt once a week or more, on the average, give yourself 1 point. The fishing must involve active work, such as rowing a boat. Sitting on the dock does not count. Hunting must include a good amount of walking and carrying equipment.

_____ 6. If, at least once a week, you participate for an hour or more in vigorous dancing like square or folk dancing, give yourself 1 point.

_____ 7. If, at least once a week, you play golf and do not use a power cart, give yourself 2 points.

_____ 8. If you often walk for exercise or recreation, give yourself 1 point.

_____ 9. If, when you are bothered by pressures at work or at home, you use exercise as a way to relax, give yourself 1 point.

_____10. If you perform calisthenics, such as sit-ups and push-ups, for at least ten minutes per session, two or more times a week, give yourself 3 points.

_____11. If you regularly perform stretching exercises, give yourself 2 points.

_____12. If you participate in active recreational sports, such as tennis or football:

   (a) About once a week, give yourself 2 points.
   (b) About twice a week, give yourself 4 points.
   (c) Three times a week or more, give yourself 7 points.

_____13. If you participate in vigorous physical activities, such as jogging or swimming for at least twenty continuous minutes per session:

   (a) About once a week, give yourself 3 points.
   (b) About twice a week, give yourself 5 points.
   (c) Three times a week or more, give yourself 10 points.

Total your points _____ .

Calculating Your Score

In order to determine your approximate level of fitness (to get a completely accurate figure would require extensive scientific testing and calculations), find where your score fits according to the following information:

☐ If you scored 0 to 5 points, your level of activity is termed *sedentary*. The amount of activity you do in a day is not adequate and usually leads to a steady deterioration in fitness.

☐ If you scored 6 to 11 points, your level of activity is termed *light activity*. This amount of activity will slow the rate of fitness loss, but it will not maintain an adequate fitness level in most persons.

☐ If you scored 12 to 20 points, your level of activity is termed *moderate activity*. This amount of activity will maintain an acceptable level of physical fitness.

☐ If you scored 21 points or more, your level of activity is termed *heavy activity*. This level of activity will maintain a high state of physical fitness.

Now that you have determined your activity level, you will need to figure how this affects the calories you spend each day for voluntary muscle activities.

☐ If your activity level is *sedentary,* you will need to add 40-50 percent to your BMR.

☐ If your activity level is *light,* add 55-65 percent.

☐ For *moderate* activity, add 65-70 percent.

☐ For *heavy* activity, add 75-100 percent.[2]

If the man we have used in our example had a desk job, he would estimate the energy he needed for voluntary muscle activities by multiplying his BMR calories per day by about 50 percent. John's BMR calories were 1,632 per day times 50 percent for his sedentary lifestyle to arrive at an additional figure of 816 calories per day.

Alice teaches physical education in a junior high school. As a result, her level of activity is *moderate*. She takes the 1,464 calories she figured her body spends for involuntary activities times 65 percent to arrive at a figure of 952 calories per day.

Calculate the approximate number of calories you spend per day on voluntary muscle activity.[2]

Total the Two Components of Energy Output

Now, total the two components together. Take the approximate amount of calories your body spends per day for basal metabolism and add to it the approximate number of calories you spend per day in voluntary muscle activity. The figure you arrive at is an estimate of the number of calories your body spends each day on energy output. If you want to maintain your current weight, this is the approximate number of calories you would need to consume as food energy. If you eat more calories than this figure, you may gain weight. If you eat fewer calories than this figure, you may lose weight.

In our example, John's BMR (or basal metabolic rate) was 1,632 calories. He adds to it the 816 calories he spends per day on voluntary activities to get a total of 2,448 calories spent each day for energy output. John will need to consume approximately 2,448 calories per day to maintain his just-reached goal weight. Alice's BMR was 1,464 calories to which she added the 952 calories spent for voluntary activity to get a total of 2,416 calories.

Factors Which Influence BMR

There are many factors which influence the BMR: age, height, growth, body composition, fever, stress, environmental temperature, fasting or starvation, malnutrition, and thyroxine. In youth, the BMR is higher; age brings less lean body mass and slows the BMR. Height is a factor; tall, thin people generally have higher BMRs. Growth affects BMR; children and pregnant women have higher BMRs. Your body composition affects the BMR because the more lean tissue, the higher the BMR. The more fat tissue, the lower the BMR. If you are running a fever, your body spends more calories trying to maintain a normal temperature and your BMR rises. Stress hormones increase the BMR. Both heat and cold raise the BMR. For example, if you are sitting in a climate-controlled building all the time, you do not spend as many calories as someone who works outside in temperature extremes. Fasting and starvation hormones lower the BMR, as does malnutrition. The thyroid hormone thyroxine is a key BMR regulator; the more thyroxine produced, the higher the BMR.

Increasing Your BMR

Were you surprised to see how many calories your body uses each day just for basal metabolic processes? You cannot do much to change this component. You can, however, change the second component—voluntary muscle activities—and spend more calories today. If you want to increase your basal metabolic rate, make moderate exercise a daily habit and eat a well-balanced diet. The *Weigh to Win* Rainbow Food Plan provides the necessary nutrients which your body needs to function properly and sustain life. Your body composition will become more lean, and your basal metabolic rate will increase as well.

Psalm 139:14 declares, "I praise You because I am fearfully and wonderfully made; Your works are wonderful, I know that full well."

In 1 Corinthians 12:12, 18, we read, "The body is a unit, though it is made up of many parts; and though all its parts are many, they form one body. . . . in fact, God has arranged the parts in the body, every one of them, just as He wanted them to be."

God has given us bodies that are complex and "wonderfully made." The Bible says He arranged all the parts just as He wanted them to be. We have a responsibility to take care of our bodies, to provide them with the nutrients needed to sustain a consistent quality of life, and exercise enough to keep them functioning properly.

FIFTEEN

Are You a Sneak Eater?

Do you nibble at salads, vegetables, and fruit in public, but stuff down a bag of potato chips as soon as you get home? Do you eat only one or two pieces of chocolate in front of others, knowing that you have a whole stash of candy bars tucked away in a drawer for later? Do you keep food hidden in the glove compartment of your car to munch on while you drive? Do you eat quickly, standing in front of the refrigerator, hoping no one will catch you? Do you eat nutritiously in front of your children to set a good example, but head for the munchies after they have gone to school?

If you have answered *yes* to any or all of these questions, you are a sneak eater. Whether you eat in secret every day or only once in a while, your sneak eating is dangerous. When you are sneak eating you are lying to yourself. It poisons your self-esteem and it is bad for your emotional health. To avoid being found out when you are sneak eating, you usually eat fast. You do not take time to savor your food, so you do not feel satisfied. When you eat fast, you are likely to eat a lot more food than you really need. It takes about twenty minutes for the "message" to get from your stomach through your nervous system to your brain that you are full. I know that I used to be able to chow down a lot of food in twenty minutes! When you eat in secret, you do not pay attention to your body's messages. Getting the food down your throat and out of sight is all that really matters.

Why Do You Sneak Eat?

Why do you find yourself sneak eating? Is it because you feel guilty about your eating habits and by sneak eating you are trying to hide the fact that your eating habits need to be changed?

By sneak eating you avoid taking responsibility for your eating habits. Sneak eating is self-deception. Somehow you think that the food you eat in secret has no calories and will not show up as a weight gain.

Sneak eating gives you a false sense of being in control. You can fix a sandwich the way *you* want it. No compromising—no worrying about someone else. No having to fix the sandwich on white bread because no one else in the family will eat rye bread —you can have it the way you want. It is a form of rebellion. It is a time when you and you alone decide what you will eat and no one else can do a thing about it. You control the situation.

Secret eating may indicate the need for time alone. Do you stay up late watching television while the rest of the family goes to bed, because you can have some time to yourself to focus entirely on your food? Some people feel that food eaten in secret tastes better than food eaten in front of others. Somehow the turkey you sneak off the bones following the big Thanksgiving dinner tastes better than the portion you had on your plate at the table. You are already full, but you just cannot stop yourself from nibbling as you clean up the kitchen. Everybody else is in the family room watching the football game. No one will ever know.

One trait all sneak eaters share is the desire to avoid responsibility for their self-destructive behavior. A major key to permanent weight loss is *ownership,* taking responsibility for your actions. Statements such as, "I don't know how I got fat —I hardly eat anything at all!" indicate that the person speaking is refusing to accept responsibility for his or her actions. It is very difficult to lose weight if you do not take responsibility for having gained it in the first place.

Overcoming Sneak Eating

How do you overcome sneak eating?

☐ First, eat openly instead of secretively. Even if you are making unwise choices, do it openly and honestly. Anything which you would eat in secret ought to be able to be eaten in front of others. Otherwise, do not eat it! You can lose weight this time and keep it off by eating openly. Come out of hiding! Ask yourself, "Who or what am I hiding from? Family members, spouse, thinner friends? The mirror?" What do you imagine these people would say if they actually caught you eating in secret? Remember, it is quite easy to project your own self-condemnation onto other people.

☐ Second, do not judge yourself harshly or promise yourself that you will never sneak food again. Unrealistic expectations often create the problem in the first place. Take a more moderate approach and get through one day at a time saying, "For today I will not eat anything in secret." If you do falter, don't give up. Remind yourself that a commitment to God does not mean you will never fail; rather, it means that you will keep on trying until you succeed.

☐ Third, speak up. First Corinthians 14:25 warns, "The secrets of his heart will be laid bare." Discuss your eating with a friend you trust, or talk to the members of your *Weigh to Win* support group. Airing problems makes them seem less serious and sets the stage for getting your eating under control.

☐ Fourth, be creatively "naughty." Let yourself be "bad" occasionally without overeating. You might splurge and buy a book in hard cover without waiting for the paperback to come out; take a nap or soak in the bathtub; take the afternoon off and play a round of golf; buy some new clothes even though you know they will be too big in a few weeks.

☐ Fifth, plan times of solitude. Do not be afraid to be alone. All solitary eating does not have to be taboo. It is possible to eat *in private* without eating in secret. Prepare a nice, healthy, *Weigh to Win* snack and then tell your family, "I am going to the bedroom to eat my snack. See you later!"

☐ Sixth, break the "I should" habit. First Peter 1:13 says, "Therefore, prepare your minds for action; be self-controlled; set your hope fully on the grace to be given you." When you spend all day working and doing chores, it is no wonder that you feel you deserve a treat by evening. But instead of merely giving in to the "I am going to reward myself with food" syndrome, prepare your mind for action.

List below all the activities you do in a typical day, everything from brushing your teeth to tucking the kids in at night.

	S/W		S/W
_____	__	_____	__
_____	__	_____	__
_____	__	_____	__
_____	__	_____	__
_____	__	_____	__
_____	__	_____	__
_____	__	_____	__
_____	__	_____	__
_____	__	_____	__
_____	__	_____	__
_____	__	_____	__

Now, go through your list and mark an "S" next to all the activities you do because you "should" do them and a "W" next to all the activities you do because you "want to" do them. Do you have a lot more "Ss" than "Ws"? Work to distribute your "W" activities more evenly throughout the day. "W" activities might include taking a walk during your lunch hour, splurging on a Saturday afternoon game of tennis, getting a facial or a manicure, or taking time to read the newspaper.

☐ Seventh, stay aware. Many sneak eaters "blank out" when they binge, as if they are in a trance to numb their feelings. Try eating in front of a mirror. Awareness leads to change.

By putting these tips into practice, you will be taking the first step toward freeing yourself from sneak eating. As with most things in life, openness—not secrecy—is the best policy.

Sixteen

Getting Control of the Urge to Eat

Before you can plan ways to change your eating habits, you must be able to describe when and how you eat. You must know the hours of the day when your appetite is most likely to get out of hand or the times your urge to eat is best under control.

We all share a common frailty—we often confuse what we would like to have done with what we actually did. The Apostle Paul said, "I do not understand what I do. For what I want to do I do not do, but what I hate I do. . . . For I have the desire to do what is good, but I cannot carry it out" (Romans 7:15, 18).

We may think that we have followed an eating plan, when really we ate much more than we intended. For instance, Charles praised himself for passing up the sweet potatoes with marshmallows on top and pumpkin pie à la mode at Thanksgiving dinner; but what about the three rolls he used to sop the greasy turkey gravy? He told himself green beans were a good choice, but he conveniently ignored the fact that they were swimming in a buttery cream sauce with french fried onion rings on top. We delude ourselves in several ways.

☐ *The Denial Delusion.* The first source of delusion is denial. We like to emphasize aspects of our behavior which please us most and play down our weaknesses. We may boast to others, "I have no problem resisting potato chips. I haven't had a potato chip in years." What we fail to mention is that every Saturday morning we go to the bakery for a sweet roll. Denial is a defense mechanism which helps maintain a positive self-image. It can be a useful tool, but when it becomes excessive it can lead to self-defeating behavior. As long as Charles denies his excesses, he will not be able to control them.

☐ *The Distraction Delusion.* Distraction is another form of delusion. Charles was distracted by the warm family feeling at the Thanksgiving dinner. When the distractions arouse emotions, the effect is even greater. Family eating traditions distract us from making healthy choices and we delude ourselves into thinking the extra pounds are not going to show up on the scale next week.

☐ *The Distortion Delusion.* The final source of delusion is distortion. People are more likely to judge their eating intake by what they think they ate than by what they actually ate. Expectation reaches out and bends experience out of shape. Keep your portion size firmly in mind and determine before eating that you will be satisfied. When you decide in advance that something will please, the food will do the job. If not, large quantities can go "down the hatch" before you realize it.

Overcoming the Three Delusions

You can defeat the three Ds if you keep written records of your eating habits. These records will help you in two ways:

☐ You will get an accurate picture of how your eating relates to your emotions.

☐ You will have the information necessary to bring poor eating habits under control just because you are aware of what is taking place.

If you try to change lifelong eating habits from where you *would like to be* instead of where you *really are,* your plans will not be very effective. Recording your eating responses will put you on guard and help you to recognize the opportunities you have to make different choices which provide you with the likelihood of remaining in control of your eating.

Keep a Record

Your record needs to be specific, simple, and written down before the eating takes place—see My Eating Record at the end of this chapter. For each hour of your day, beginning with the usual hour you wake up, and continuing hour by hour for the entire twenty-four hour period, rate the level of your urge to eat from 0 to 4 with 0 being *no* desire.

Mark a 1 if you feel your urge to eat is true, physical hunger. This should occur only if it has been at least four to six hours after a satisfying meal.

Mark a 2 if the desire to eat may be physical; however, it could be a psychological or learned response to food.

Mark a 3 if you feel a moderate desire to eat but know you are not physically in need of food. At this stage, you are able to shift your attention away from food by changing your focus.

Mark a 4 if the desire to eat is very strong and you know it is not a physical need for food. At this stage, you try to put food out of your mind but find your thoughts constantly turning to food.

A desire to eat is often a response to feelings such as boredom, frustration, tension, and proximity to food. If you are exposed to these cues, you may eat even though your physical urge to eat is very low. It is important that you train yourself to differentiate between eating which is motivated by true, physical need for food and an internally triggered, learned desire for food which is due to external events.

Recording your eating pattern helps you to focus on the vital question, "Is this food really necessary?" By asking this question before you eat, you give yourself the chance to bring the desire to eat under control.

As you record the overall level of your desire to eat hour by hour, mark *Yes* if you did eat, and *No* if you did not. Leave room for some notes to record what action you plan to take, if the desire to eat reaches the 2 to 4 level. Write down the times you were successful; give yourself a written "pat on the back," and give the Lord Jesus praise for His help and strength.

Keep this record every day for at least a week. Through this record you will learn that there are times when you are truly free from the desire to eat and other times when the desire to eat seems to dominate your life. These are the times when decisions can be made to help you achieve self-control.

Jesus realized the importance of the need for food when He spoke to the 5,000 people and told His disciples, "They do not need to go away. You give them something to eat" (Matthew 14:16). He blessed the healthy loaves and fishes, and "They all ate and were satisfied, and the disciples picked up twelve basketfuls of broken pieces that were left over" (v. 20). We can eat and be satisfied too, if we will ask the Lord to help us become aware of a desire to eat which is psychological or a learned response instead of a desire to eat which is truly physical hunger.

MY EATING RECORD

Day of the week:

Time*	Level of urge to eat	Did you eat? Yes	No	Action taken or action you plan to take
6–7 AM				
7–8 AM				
8–9 AM				
9–10 AM				
10–11 AM				
11–12 PM				
12–1 PM				
1–2 PM				
2–3 PM				
3–4 PM				
4–5 PM				
5–6 PM				
6–7 PM				
7–8 PM				
8–9 PM				
9–10 PM				
10–11 PM				
11–12 AM				
12–6 AM				

Mark 0 if you feel no urge to eat.

Mark 1 if you feel hunger and believe that it is a physically motivated urge to eat.

Mark 2 if you feel the urge to eat is somewhere between a physically and psychologically motivated urge to eat.

Mark 3 if you feel a mild urge to eat and know that you are not in physical need of food.

Mark 4 if you feel a strong urge to eat and know that you are not in physical need of food.

*Change the hours of the day as necessary on the Eating Record, to accommodate your unique schedule.

SEVENTEEN

Controlling Your Appetite While Boosting Your Spirit (Exercise and Weight Loss)

There was a time when the sidewalks of cities everywhere were crowded. Now walkers and bike riders are the exception and not the rule. Backyards or empty lots were once filled with children and adults "playing catch" in the early evening or "shooting a few baskets." Now many spend their Sundays watching football on television and the parks are just for "those health nuts." We used to sharpen our pencils, chop our ice, and open our cans by hand. Now these and dozens of other minor jobs are done with marvelous electronic inventions.

In short, we will spare no expense and will apply the height of creativity to be able to push a button rather than move an arm, to sit instead of stand, or to ride rather than walk. There is now no task too minor to warrant calling upon a machine to do the job for us and no trip too short to hold us back from climbing into the family car. My own children would beg, "Mom, it's just not cool to walk to school—won't you take us? If you don't take us, the other kids will make fun of us." As a caring mom, of course, I did not want my children to be made fun of, so I dutifully loaded them up and took them to school.

Because of this energy-sparing way of life, Americans have become sedentary and soft. Our bellies have broadened and our stamina has decreased. We huff and puff climbing a few stairs. Yet, it is not at all unusual to read statements like, "Exercise? You would have to climb to the top of Mount Everest to lose one single pound," or "If you are trying to walk your weight off, forget it! You would have to walk from dawn to dusk to get rid of one pound of fat." An ad for a weight loss organization touted, "No Exercise." Statements such as these are music to the ears of exercise-loathing individuals who use them to justify their lack of activity.

The Role of Activity in Weight Control

While some authorities question the role of activity in weight control, the Food and Nutrition Board of the National Research Council clearly recognizes its importance and recommends 300 more calories per day for men and women who engage in *moderate* activity, and 600–900 more calories for those who engage in *heavy* activity. It therefore stands to reason that anyone who holds caloric levels constant and increases their level of activity would have to burn fat stores to fuel this extra effort.

What does this mean for Sam and Sue who are trying to use activity to burn off extra calories? Assuming that they both weigh 150 pounds, they would have to spend about seventeen minutes walking briskly to burn up the calories in a banana. A donut would require about twenty minutes of walking. An ice cream soda is worth about a forty-nine minute walk. A generous helping of strawberry shortcake would keep them on the sidewalk for about seventy-seven minutes. Does this sound like a whole lot of work for a small reward? Well, let us take another look. If Sam and Sue took a thirty-minute walk, they would burn 150 calories. If they would walk five days a week for a year, and if their food intake stayed the same throughout the year, they would burn approximately 39,000 extra calories, enough to shed about eleven pounds in twelve months, twenty-two pounds in two years. If Sam and Sue weighed more than 150 pounds, their reward would be even greater. Therefore, the longer you spend at it, and the heavier you are, the more calories you will burn for the effort.

The Benefits of Exercise

The benefit of exercise continues long after you sit down to rest. The rate of metabolism stays higher for several hours after a vigorous workout. This means that hours after the activity ends, your body may burn extra fat.

Besides the obvious weight loss benefits of activity, exercise can also improve the health of the heart and circulatory system by helping to prevent the buildup of extra cholesterol in the bloodstream. It can help you feel better mentally and emotionally in several important ways.

☐ It reduces your level of tension and stress.

☐ It helps you to sleep better.

☐ It sharpens your concentration.

☐ It betters your mood.

☐ It reduces your appetite.

☐ It improves your self-confidence.

Tension manifests itself physically by keeping muscles taut and rigid. As you work out your tension with activity, your muscles relax and sleep comes more easily. When you feel rested, you are able to concentrate on your work and meet the challenges of everyday living. When your day goes well, you feel more positive as well. When you feel more relaxed and more enthusiastic, you may find that your urge to over-eat is reduced. You are also more likely to make healthy food choices when your mind is clear and your body is rested.

A real danger time is when you are physically or mentally tired. Even though you are bone weary, if you will make yourself get out and just take a little walk, you may come back better able to cope with the evening ahead and the food choices you need for good health.

Exercise Decreases Appetite and Increases Self-Esteem

Instead of increasing your appetite, light to moderate activity *decreases* it. If activity helps you keep control of your urge to eat, then you feel better about yourself and more positive about the future.

Increased activity also builds self-esteem in two ways. First, when you do something active you are doing something for all the world to see. You are showing others that you are acting for your own well-being. Second, you are keeping a commitment to yourself and to your health. You feel good knowing that you have finished a job well done. Matthew 25:21 says, "His master replied, 'Well done, good and faithful servant! You have been faithful with a few things; I will put you in charge of many things. Come and share your master's happiness!' "

When I am out walking, I imagine the Lord looking down at me from the beautiful blue sky with a big, loving smile, saying, "Well done!" He knows how difficult exercise has always been for me. I was terrible in physical education in school. A fear of water kept me from enjoying swimming. I was never quick enough or muscular enough to excel at sports. My pear-shaped body keeps me from looking good in shorts, no matter how thin I am. To overcome all these negative feelings and get out there and exercise is a real achievement for me.

Find Your Path to Fitness

Through the years I have tried various kinds of exercise. My overweight body just could not get into the contortions most aerobic instructors in their flashy spandex leotards demonstrated. Deep muscle exercises aggravated my back problem. Climbing stairs stirred up the arthritis in my knee. Calisthenics were boring and I did not have the stamina to run. I was not coordinated enough to follow the dance steps of some jazz-style exercises. A tight budget made joining a health club prohibitive. I could have let all of these negatives keep me from doing any type of exercise but just as I had searched for a way of eating which I could do for the rest of my life, I knew that I had to find a way of exercising which I could do for the rest of my life.

Walking was the answer for me. When the weather or time of day prohibits walking out of doors, an electronic treadmill takes its place. Travel and work schedules sometimes interfere, but I have really learned to enjoy putting a cassette tape in a tape player and taking off out the door for a forty-five-minute walk.

You can find a way of exercising which fits you. If you enjoy aerobics, then do it! If you can do stair climbing and enjoy the challenge of increasing the number of steps you can climb each time, then go for it! If a nice morning swim invigorates you the whole day, then do it! Just as each of us is unique in God's sight, each of us must find the method of exercise which is appropriate for us, individually.

NOTE: Please be aware that an increase in activity should not be undertaken without specific medical approval, if you are pregnant, or if you have suffered any cardiovascular stress, including hypertension and heart attacks. If you have diabetes, electrolyte imbalances, anemia, varicose veins, and related medical problems, plan any activity with great care. If you are very overweight or out of shape, a rapid increase in activity could lead to joint problems or other forms of physical stress. It is important to consult your doctor before you start to exercise.

Exercise Excuses

Do you have a case of *Can't* or *Won't?* People often make excuses when it comes to exercise. They think it is going to make them too hungry. But to the contrary, light to moderate activity has been shown to decrease appetite. If you feel hungry, it is probably just because you have learned to reward yourself with food for doing something you really did not want to do. Remember from your childhood the number of times you may have been told to "sit still" or "be quiet," and then you were rewarded with a piece of candy for your unwilling compliance? You really did not want to sit still or be quiet, but you learned that if you did, you would be rewarded with a food treat. Those learned behaviors carry over into adult life in so many ways that we often do not even recognize them for what they are—learned behaviors which need to be overcome with the Lord's help.

Many people think physical activity means vigorous exercise with sweat seeping out of every pore and sore aching muscles for days afterward. *Physical activity means any effort to move your body around more than is your normal pattern.* You can be physically active without getting out of breath, overheated, or even changing out of your street clothes.

Another excuse frequently offered is that exercise is dull. If you do not like doing knee bends and toe touches, you are usually not going to continue the exercise long enough to be effective. There are dozens of activities which can be useful to you. It is important to find an activity which fits your individual preferences in order for you to be able to make a commitment which will mean long-term success.

Some people do not want to draw public attention to themselves, but many exercises can be done in the privacy of home or in unobtrusive ways in public places. For example, climbing stairs at the office instead of taking the elevator can be helpful. There are a variety of exercise tapes available for persons of all shapes and sizes—even tapes for persons who use wheelchairs, crutches, and braces which hinder activity.

Another activity "won't" comes from the belief that any worthwhile activity requires too much planning and too many people. If baseball is your game, you need enough others to make two teams. If you play tennis, you will need to find a court. But there are many activities which you may do "solo," such as swimming, bicycling, ice skating, rope jumping, or hitting a tennis ball against a wall. Walking or climbing stairs requires no companions, no equipment, and is free!

Finally, the most common excuse for avoiding exercise is simply that it involves change. Increased activity means using muscles which have been in mothballs for years; it also means getting in touch with your body in ways which you may not have experienced before. Above all, it means developing new attitudes; this may be the hardest change of all.

Using Energy in Everyday Activities

You need to find ways to use more energy in everyday activities.

☐ If you normally sit while talking on the telephone, try standing.

☐ If you ask others to bring the dishes to you so that you can wash them, get the dishes yourself.

☐ If you usually watch TV after dinner, take a twenty-minute walk instead.

☐ If you clean the basement and garage only once a year, think about bringing them up to snuff more often.

☐ If you normally ride the bus to work or school, try boarding the bus a stop or two farther from your home and get off a stop or two from your office or school.

☐ If you normally ride the elevator, use the stairs instead.

☐ If you usually sit at your desk or in a staff lunchroom for a break, try using the time to walk the hallways.

☐ If you usually eat in the staff cafeteria, try walking several blocks to a restaurant instead.

☐ If you rely on others to bring work to you, see if you can find ways to fetch the work yourself.

The watchword is to do as much as you can yourself, relying as little as possible on others.

Plan Larger Activities

Besides these small increases in activity, it is wise to engage in a larger activity three to five times a week. You might plan a walk, gradually increasing your time, distance walked, or walking speed. In working out a plan for personal activity, it is a good idea to follow some specific rules after receiving your doctor's okay.

☐ Choose an activity that fits you, not one which you think you "should" select.

☐ Plan specific ways to increase your activity every single day.

☐ Make a commitment to a moderate exercise program to be done three to five times a week.

☐ If you can, find someone to join in your activities, but always be prepared to go it alone.

☐ Start slow and easy, gradually increasing your speed and endurance.

Make backup plans for bad weather and days you may have to "go it alone." If you walk twenty minutes a day, do not let a snowy or rainy day give you an excuse—climb steps twenty times instead. If you plan to play tennis, be ready for a brisk walk around the park if your partner does not show up.

Now that you know the essentials, the next move is yours. Make that move now! The longer you wait, the less likely it is that you will act. Plan your program, writing down how you are going to achieve your goal (see next page) and then follow through.

Let us not be like the people in Jesus' parable in Luke 14:18, "But they all alike began to make excuses." Instead, let us look to Galatians 6:4. "Each one should test his own actions. Then he can take pride in himself, without comparing himself to somebody else."

Steps to Achieve My Activity Goals

1. _____

2. _____

3. _____

4. _____

5. _____

EIGHTEEN

Yes! You Can!
Guidelines for Dining Out

Have you ever been on one of those weight loss programs where you could not go out for dinner with a friend because there was nothing on the menu you were allowed to eat? Do you think that you cannot possibly lose weight because your work or lifestyle requires that you eat out a majority of your meals?

When you are following the sensible, healthy way of eating taught by the *Weigh to Win* Rainbow Food Plan, it is possible to eat out *and* lose weight or maintain your weight loss. In some cases, it may be easier to eat in a restaurant than to eat at home, once you know what choices to make and how to ask for your food to be prepared. Unless you make the mistake of going to an all-you-can-eat smorgasbord (talk about willpower!), the restaurant only serves you a certain portion of food. At home, you may be tempted to eat seconds and thirds!

For some people, eating out is a once-in-a-while treat. For others it is a frequent necessity. Whichever it is for you, these guidelines will help you to make the best choices possible so that you are able to succeed with the *Weigh to Win Weight Management System.*

Full-Service Restaurants

Most restaurants have a varied menu. Thus, your food plan should not be hindered by the selections offered. If you have a question about the ingredients of a menu item, be sure to ask the waiter or waitress about it before ordering. Make up your mind in advance to choose only menu items permitted by the *Weigh to Win* Rainbow Food Plan.

☐ *Meats/Protein.* When ordering meats, the best choice is broiled, baked, or roasted meat (fish, chicken, or steak). Although a broiled hamburger is allowed on the *Weigh to Win* Rainbow Food Plan, it is best to avoid eating hamburger frequently, even if it is broiled, because of its variable fat content. If hamburger is 85 percent lean or leaner, it is acceptable as long as it is 100 percent beef and is not fried. Ask that any meat be prepared without fat and that fat be trimmed before cooking, if possible. Be wary of the term "grilled" as it may actually mean that the meat is cooked on a flat grill which is the same as frying. If it says "char-grilled," that usually means the meat has been broiled on a rack.

Until you learn to "eyeball" portion sizes, ask for the cooked weight of the meat. If the server only knows the raw weight, consider the cooked weight to be about one-fourth to one-third less than the raw weight, to allow for shrinkage during cooking. The rule of thumb is that eight ounces of raw meat shrinks to six ounces cooked; six ounces of raw meat shrinks to four ounces cooked; four ounces of raw meat shrinks to three ounces cooked; and three ounces of raw meat shrinks to two ounces cooked.

☐ *Vegetables/Salads.* Ask that your vegetable serving be prepared without margarine, butter, or fat. Do not eat sauces which contain flour, cream, milk, eggs, or cheese, such as hollandaise or cheese sauce.

Vegetable salads are usually a good choice with a small amount of dressing. Request that salad dressings be brought "on the side" and that croutons be left off. Ask if the salad is all vegetables. Many times egg or cheese is served on the salad, and each adds protein. Beware of tuna, chicken, or seafood salads which may come coated with mayonnaise. Fresh fruit salads are a good choice as long as they are not in a sugar syrup or coated with mayonnaise, sour cream, or whipped cream. Pasta salads may be a good choice unless they are soaking in an oily Italian dressing! Taco salads are not a good choice because they usually come in a deep fried tortilla shell. Refried beans often contain lard, and the taco meat is generally fried and not broiled. A typical taco salad with salsa instead of sour cream is about **950** calories!

☐ *Breads/Starchy Vegetables.* Crackers, hard rolls, or plain bread are usually available. Limit your choices to the amount of bread which you are allowed on the *Weigh to Win* Rainbow Food Plan. If you choose potato, corn, or green peas, remember that starchy vegetables are counted as bread servings on the food plan. Commercially prepared rolls, biscuits, or cornbread may contain a high amount of saturated fat. An occasional indulgence is acceptable, as long as you understand that a one-ounce roll counts as one bread serving. The typical restaurant baked potato weighs about six ounces and would count as two bread servings. Just eat half and take the other half home! Ask for your baked potato "dry" or with margarine "on the side."

☐ *Fats.* If butter is served to you, ask if margarine is available. Butter is not allowed on the *Weigh to Win* Rainbow

Food Plan because of its cholesterol content. Regular salad dressings are almost pure fat and should be used sparingly.

Avoid the high-fat sour cream, margarine, or butter which may be served automatically on your potato if you do not ask for it dry.

☐ *Beverages.* For a refreshing beverage, skim milk, tomato juice, or fruit juice may be selected in allowed amounts. Other choices include coffee, tea, or diet soda in moderate amounts. Always have plenty of water served with your meal. A slice of lemon in the water adds a nice touch.

☐ *Dessert.* Give up dessert? Not necessarily. Fruit, either unsweetened or fresh, is usually the best selection. Ask if sugar-free gelatin is available. A good trick for those restaurants which automatically give you a sundae dish for free soft-serve ice cream is to fill it with allowed amounts of cottage cheese and fresh fruit from the salad bar — it looks good and tastes good too! Tell yourself that when you get home you will have some dietetic ice cream or a *Weigh to Win* dessert. Until then, drink another glass of water. The other desserts are "just not worth it."

Fast-food Restaurants

To choose a fast-food restaurant, you need to keep food preparation firmly in mind, and even then healthy food choices are quite limited. Fast food may mean *fat* food if you are not choosing wisely. A few franchises broil much of their meat, while most of the others simply grill the meats on a flat surface, cooking the meat in its own grease. As we said before, watch out for the term "grilled" — it may mean fried on a flat grill. Char-grilled usually means grilled on a rack; this is an acceptable method of food preparation.

☐ *Meats/Protein.* If you choose a fast-food roast beef sandwich, remove any visible fat. Order the regular or small size, not the super size. If lean roast beef is not available, hamburgers which are broiled are an alternative. Again, do not order the giant size Just order a regular hamburger. Some fast-food restaurants offer broiled or roasted chicken sandwiches. These are usually healthy choices as long as all the skin is removed and there is no breading. Be sure to ask that mayonnaise or other salad dressings be left off, or they will automatically appear on your sandwich. You may want to ask for mustard, instead. Do not choose fried chicken, fried fish, or tenderloin, even if it is with the intention of removing the skin or batter. Removing the skin or batter does not remove enough of the fat to be acceptable.

The first time you order, take your meal home. Weigh the meat so that you will know what portion size you are consuming, for the next time you order. Many fast-food restaurants now list nutrition information through pamphlets or posters on the wall. This information can be very helpful in making the best choices. It may also surprise you to find out what poor food choices you have consumed in years past.

Some fast-food restaurants offer a baked chicken or baked fish dinner. If the dinner comes with coleslaw, ask for a tossed salad instead. Beware that rice or vegetable accompaniments may contain added fat.

Eating at a pizza place does not mean that you have to order pizza! Many Italian-style restaurants offer pasta dishes, sandwiches, or a salad bar which would be better choices. Do not eat too many of the tempting breadsticks!

☐ *Vegetables/Salads.* A variety of salads is available at many fast-food establishments, but beware of the large packet of fattening dressing served with the healthy salad. Use only a small portion of the dressing and throw the remainder away or take it home and refrigerate it for later use. Ask that croutons and bacon be left off of your salad. Cheese, eggs, and meat add protein and calories. Omit these items unless you include them as part of your daily protein servings. If you order a chicken salad, be sure the chicken is not fried, breaded, or in a mayonnaise base. Take the salad home the first time and weigh the chicken so that you know the amount of protein you are consuming.

☐ *Breads/Starchy Vegetables.* Leave french fries alone, even if they are fried in "no cholesterol" shortening. Fried mushrooms, fried zucchini, or fried cheese sticks which are batter dipped and deep fat fried are not healthy choices.

The buns on regular-size fast-food sandwiches generally count as two bread servings. If you have the servings coming to you on your food plan, go right ahead. Otherwise, you may only want to eat half the bun.

Baked potatoes are sometimes available at fast-food restaurants, but I have seen a whole ladle full of melted butter or margarine poured on the potato before the cheese and healthy broccoli were added. Ask for a potato with *no* butter.

Saltine crackers are usually available and are a good choice. Avoid other types of crackers which may have a high fat content.

☐ *Dessert.* Fresh fruit is an excellent choice for a refreshing and satisfying dessert, but it is seldom available in fast-food restaurants unless it is on a salad bar.

Fried pies, ice cream, ice milk, turnovers, cookies, and frozen yogurt are not healthy choices, due to the fat and/or sugar content.

☐ *Beverages.* You may choose coffee, tea, or diet soft drinks as a beverage, as long as you drink them in moderation. Fruit drinks are not a healthy choice unless they are unsweetened and made from 100 percent fruit juice. Lemonade and orangeade are full of sugar and are to be avoided. Do not choose milkshakes or slush drinks. Unsweetened orange juice is often available and is a good choice. Your very best choice is *water.*

Dining Out Successfully

A good rule of thumb is, "Do not eat it unless you are certain that you know what the ingredients are, what the portion size is, and how it is prepared." And, do not be afraid to *ask.* Restaurants want your business, and they are usually very cooperative about serving your food as you ask. If the restaurant does not cooperate, vote with your feet and don't go there again.

I have found that I am able to eat out virtually anywhere because I have learned to make the best choices available. When you are standing in line at the fast-food restaurant staring at the menu overhead with its assortment of cookies, shakes, and ice cream, it takes a conscious effort and decision to disregard the foods which would not be healthy choices and concentrate on the foods which are better. When the server at your favorite full-service restaurant offers dessert before the check is brought to your table, or when the dessert cart is put right next to you, you must tell the Lord that you choose a healthy body but that you need Him to give you the strength to resist. He promises in Matthew 28:20, "And surely I am with you always, to the very end of the age."

God gave Adam and Eve a great variety of foods to enjoy. He warned them of one tree which would cause them to surely die. "And the Lord God commanded the man, 'You are free to eat from any tree in the garden; but you must not eat from the tree of the knowledge of good and evil, for when you eat of it you will surely die" (Genesis 2:16-17). God has given us a great variety of wonderful, healthy foods to choose from on this earth. Let us make good choices and turn away from the few foods which are not good choices for our bodies, the foods which have caused us to be overweight, the foods which can lead to serious health problems.

Will you ever be able to eat that dessert? An occasional indulgence is not harmful, once you have reached your weight loss goals and have learned to control your food choices rather than letting them control you. Once in a while, I will have a piece of pie or some ice cream after a sensible restaurant meal, using amounts allowed by the *Weigh to Win* Lifetime Maintenance Program. But, until you reach your weight loss goals, such foods are detours on your journey and they are just not worth it.

Yes! You can dine out. Just choose wisely!

NINETEEN
Children and Weight Loss

All you have to do is look around to see that the number of overweight children and teenagers is increasing. A lifestyle of fast food and Nintendo games frequently results in a high fat diet and little opportunity for exercise.

When I was a child we always had a garden. I was exposed to and was strongly encouraged to eat a large variety of vegetables. We would can gallons of green beans, bushels of beets, copious amounts of carrots, and what seemed like tons of tomatoes. Then we would freeze all of the sweet corn, peas, broccoli, asparagus, and cauliflower that we could pick or purchase from the local produce farms. Mom would haul my two brothers and me to the strawberry patch, blueberry patch, and apple and peach orchards, where we were taught to "pick clean"—hot sun, mosquitoes, and all. At the time, this was not fun; however, the "fruits of our labor" tasted wonderful all winter long. As I grew older I came to appreciate the value of working together as a family to "put up" food for the winter.

I feel sorry for the children of today who do not know what it is like to go out into a garden, pick a pod of peas, and taste their raw sweetness. Some children have never tasted a red, juicy, vine-ripened Indiana tomato. There is nothing so delicious as corn on the cob, picked and in the pot within minutes of the pickin'. Instead, busy lifestyles and the push of commercial marketing often make the limited variety available in fast-food restaurants or convenience foods the norm in many households.

If you have an overweight child, I would encourage you to consult a registered dietitian and a physician for help. Never try to put a child under fifteen years of age on any type of reduced-calorie diet without professional help. *Never* put a child on a diet meant for an adult, since a child's nutritional needs are very different. Unless a child is grossly overweight, changing the way *you* eat may be all that is needed for your child to start slimming down.

As parents, we have a responsibility to learn what our children need nutritionally and then to do our best to present the food to them in a positive way which encourages normal eating and adequate nutrition. The menu below is from a mother of a five-year-old child who thought she was feeding her child nutritiously.

Breakfast:	One-fourth cup of cereal with one-half cup of whole milk; unpeeled apple slices.
Lunch:	Bologna sandwich with one slice bologna on two slices of whole wheat bread; one cup of whole milk; one bag of pretzels.
Supper:	Two chicken drumsticks (fried); twenty french fries; twelve ounce can of carbonated beverage; one dinner roll; one-half cup of gelatin with whipped topping.
Snack:	Four chocolate sandwich cookies.

The following shows how this menu met, exceeded, or fell below the U.S. Recommended Daily Allowances of just a sampling of the nutrients needed by the typical five-year-old child.

Protein	259% of RDA	- higher than necessary
Vitamin A	32% of RDA	- too low
Thiamin	129% of RDA	- adequate
Riboflavin	150% of RDA	- adequate
Folacin	60% of RDA	- too low
Vitamin C	52% of RDA	- too low
Calcium	81% of RDA	- marginal
Iron	93% of RDA	- marginal
Zinc	88% of RDA	- marginal[3]

Imagine how much worse this would be if the child skipped breakfast or if more sugary foods took the place of more nourishing ones. Many parents give their child a multiple vitamin each day and expect this to make up for the deficit, but this is a second-rate substitute for obtaining the needed nutrients from foods eaten on a daily basis.

Our Learned Behaviors Affect Our Families

Besides learning accurate nutrition information, we must stop the vicious cycle of learned behaviors which have caused us as adults to be overweight, and which may be affecting our entire family. When you have children, you not only have to work to overcome your own learned behaviors, but you also have to be conscious of the fact that you may be repeating history. As a child, if you were given a cookie when you fell down and got hurt, you may hear yourself saying, "Here, Traci, this will make you feel better." What you were taught and what you are teaching your child is that food is the answer for pain, sadness, and hurts in life.

Have you found yourself saying, "No ice cream until you

finish your carrots"? Offering dessert as a reward is probably the way you were taught. If you prepare a low fat, low sugar dessert and serve it at the same time that the rest of the meal is put on the table, your child will not learn to associate dessert with the end of a meal. Let the child eat the dessert whenever he or she wishes. Offering dessert as a reward only encourages the child to overeat twice—once to finish the required food to earn the dessert and then the dessert itself.

If your child is very young, present the food in a manner that a child with immature coordination can easily handle. Finger foods or foods cut into small pieces are more likely to be eaten than food which the child has to work hard to eat.

Older children will respond more favorably to a new food or to food prepared in a different way if your attitude is positive and convincing. If you or your spouse complain about the food, do not expect Jimmy to eat it with enthusiasm.

Involving older children in the shopping, meal preparation, and decision-making process provides opportunities for them to feel more in control of their food choices and also is a learning experience. I took my children to the store and told them that they could choose any cereal they wanted as long as it had five grams or less of sucrose on the label. We made a game of it, but I knew they were learning to read labels. I allowed them to be a part of the decision-making process within the guidelines of what I knew to be best for the health of our family. Because I was consistent with the guidelines, they knew not to even ask for a sugary cereal. When nutrition is taught and explained to older children in a way that is interesting, the battle of getting them to eat well is half won.

A couple of years ago, a photographer from our local small-town newspaper snapped a picture of my daughter eating her lunch from a Kentucky Fried Chicken box under a tree at the high school. Local *Weigh to Win* members got a chuckle out of this because the choice was not what they expected from my child. I really do not worry about what my children eat when they are away from home. I put no demands or unreasonable requirements on them, such as forbidding them to eat anything with sugar in it. Children being children, such impositions would only encourage them to find a way to eat such foods and be sneaky about it. I want my children to be able to openly talk about what they eat, and I do not want food to be a major issue in their lives. If we are not careful, we can make food such an issue that we, and our children, lose perspective. Food is merely fuel for our bodies. It is important that we give our bodies the best grade and blend of fuel available in order for our bodies to function properly. Having a piece of candy once in a while is not a life or death matter, unless there are special health problems such as diabetes.

Take Responsibility for What You Feed Your Children

I have fulfilled my responsibility to my children by seeing that they have nutritious, balanced meals when they are at home and by teaching them what they need to know to make decisions concerning their own health for the rest of their lives. The refrigerator is kept stocked with fruits and vegetables for healthy after-school snacks. My daughter enjoys coming home and making several servings of rice for a snack which is considerably better than a candy bar. My son is in the teenage "can't-fill-him-up" stage and eats us out of house and home. At least I know that what he is eating at home is good for him and that he is not filling up on empty calories and junk food. A schoolmate of my daughter was surprised to learn that we do not keep potato chips in the house; she could not imagine living without them! Sometimes we will have a pizza delivered or stop for an ice cream cone, but not often. With this kind of nutrition emphasis in our home and the help of a healthy metabolism, both of my children have been spared from the weight problem I had at their age.

If your child is under fifteen years of age and has been diagnosed by your physician as being overweight, you can do wonders just by cooking *Weigh to Win* meals. Take out your portion and let your family have what they want of the rest. Keep your attitude about eating healthy positive. Consider it an adventure to experiment with new foods and new recipes. Make your meals colorful. Serving white fish, cauliflower, and a potato may be nutritious, but it has no color appeal. Colorful carrots, broccoli, or beets would give the meal more eye appeal. And don't forget garnishes. A slice of orange, lemon, tomato, or a parsley sprig makes a plate or platter look delicious. A fresh fruit dessert looks and tastes wonderful. A dish of sugar-free banana pudding with a slice of kiwi on top is sure to please.

If you are eating out with your children, guide them in making wise choices. You might say, "Karen, the baked chicken or broiled fish dinners would be good choices. If you are not very hungry, there is a cottage cheese and fresh fruit plate. Which would you like?" In this way, you allow them to make a choice but within appropriate guidelines. Use menu choices as opportunities to discuss why some foods are not healthy choices. If fast food is your choice, again give your children the options available within your knowledgeable guidelines.

Forcing your children to eat is a no-win situation. In the past, I insisted that my children at least taste a new food. Usually their minds were made up that they were not going to like it, and the screwed-up face with the "Ugh—this is terrible!" came out before the taste sensors on the tongue could possibly have registered "good" or "bad." If your children refuse to eat a certain food, do not assume that they will never eat it. Try it again in a few weeks or months. Tastes change. Moods change. Minds change.

Constantly reinforce the fact that you are trying to teach your children nutritious choices because you love them and because you want them to have the best chance at a healthy life. If you did not care about them, it would not matter what they ate—but you do care! Children do not think about the fact that the way they are eating right now may very well determine how long they live and how healthy they will be when they reach old age. You will probably not convince them of this because their young, growing bodies appear to be so healthy, even though their diet may be poor.

Share these Scripture verses with your child when the two of you are having a quiet time together:

> Do you not know that your body is a temple of the Holy Spirit, who is in you, whom you have received from God? You are not your own; you were bought at a price. Therefore honor God with your body (1 Corinthians 6:19-20).
>
> For You created my inmost being; You knit me together in my mother's womb. I praise You because I am fearfully and wonderfully made; Your works are wonderful, I know that full well (Psalm 139:13-14).

Our bodies are wonderfully made and, since the body is a temple of the Holy Spirit, we have a responsibility to honor God by taking the best possible care of it. God put wonderful foods on this earth to enjoy. His foods are designed to make our bodies function "wonderfully." We need to do what we can to honor God with the foods we eat.

Parents, please do not use these Scripture verses to bring condemnation if your child eats a cookie. You accomplish much more with compassion than condemnation. Showing that you understand why your child would want that cookie, and sympathizing with them because you too know how difficult it is to resist certain foods, will get you much farther than showing how disappointed you are.

Eating Healthy Is a Family Affair

Just as it is nearly impossible for a father to sit with a cigarette in his hand and command his son not to smoke, so is it impossible for you to eat unhealthy foods in front of your child and expect that child to be strong and resist. Your example must follow your words. This is a family project. If your spouse will not cooperate, or a brother or sister insists on bringing home unhealthy foods, the overweight child has little chance of overcoming the weight problem.

If your child had leukemia and needed a bone marrow transplant, everyone in your family would band together, have their blood tested, and help in any way they could. Helping overweight children to lose weight, or teaching normal weight children how to handle food so that they do not have a weight problem in later life, requires the family to band together in love and support.

Proverbs 22:6 promises, "Train a child in the way he should go, and when he is old he will not turn from it." Teach your child how to make wise food choices through thoughts (having a positive attitude), actions (being a good example yourself), and deeds (providing healthy food choices).

TWENTY

The Day My Wall Came Tumbling Down

Now Jericho was tightly shut up because of the Israelites. No one went out and no one came in.

Then the Lord said to Joshua, "See, I have delivered Jericho into your hands, along with its king and its fighting men. March around the city once with all the armed men. Do this for six days. Have seven priests carry trumpets of rams' horns in front of the ark. On the seventh day, march around the city seven times, with the priests blowing their trumpets. When you hear them sound a long blast on the trumpets, have all the people give a loud shout; then the wall of the city will collapse and the people will go up, every man straight in" (Joshua 6:1-5).

What has you walled in? Is it a destructive or harmful habit? Is it a wall of fear, an inferiority complex, or doubt that God's promises are true? Is it a feeling of frustration, as if you are "banging your head against a wall" when it comes to your weight loss battle?

What is your wall which seems impossible to penetrate? "See, I have delivered Jericho into your hands," said God, but Joshua could not see it. To him the wall of Jericho looked just as impossible and foreboding as ever. Only through the eyes of faith could Joshua follow through with what he had to do.

When I started my weight loss journey on March 17, 1986, the wall of fat I had around me seemed impossible and foreboding. I thought, "Why am I even thinking about trying to lose weight? I am just going to fail again." I was so afraid. Somehow, I had just enough faith to believe that if God could deliver great and mighty Jericho into the hands of the Israelites, somehow He could help me get rid of my wall of fat.

Perhaps you are on the *outside* of a wall and cannot find your way *in*. Maybe you are standing before a wall of impossibility. Do you find yourself in an impossible situation in your personal life, with your job, with your business, or your finances? Do you see your weight as a wall which seems impossible to surmount? There are steps to take to see that your wall tumbles down, just like the wall of Jericho.

You Have to Do Your Part

You will notice in the Scripture that the people had to do their part to make the wall come down. God could bring the wall down all by Himself, but He wants us to cooperate with Him. God could take an unhealthy, fattening meal out of our hands if He chose to do so. Instead He has given us a will and a mind of our own. Doing our part and making better choices will help our wall of fat to come down.

When I started losing weight the *Weigh to Win* way, I knew that I had to do the work. I had to make the best food choices—God was not going to make them for me. To be successful, it was going to take cooperation, and I was willing to do my part. I knew it was not going to be easy. I had a lot to learn. "God, teach me," I prayed.

You Must Have Self-Control

The Israelites had to show self-control. They were given specific instructions by God to accomplish the task.

☐ First, they had to move. They were told to march! They had to take action, but there was a definite plan. I am reasonably sure that they must have had to resist the temptation to go for a ladder and try to scale the wall on their own without the Lord's help. It probably seemed like a faster way too. Sometimes fad diets seem like a faster way for us too.

☐ Second, they could not be distracted. Surely they felt like they were going in circles all the time and not getting anywhere. Have you ever felt that way concerning your weight loss? It is easy to get distracted from your weight loss plan. If you get your eyes off of your goal, even for a minute, the distraction can be disastrous.

Sometimes I allowed myself to become distracted during my weight loss journey. In times past, if I became distracted I just gave up, admitting failure. Throughout my weight loss this time, I did not allow very many distractions. When I did give in and eat an ice cream treat, I let God know that I was not giving up. Sure, I was mad at myself for getting distracted, but I put the distraction behind me, regained my focus, and started right back on the *Weigh to Win* Rainbow Food Plan.

☐ Third, they were probably heckled. How silly the Israelites must have looked marching around that wall again and again. I can just picture the citizens of Jericho peering down from the top of the wall, laughing at the Israelites, and jeering at their futile plight. Some probably even tried to bribe the Israelites to get them to quit marching.

The Israelite people may have been embarrassed that they were in the situation in the first place. The Israelites were a proud people. Here they were, marching around this highly fortified city, with no weapons—just some trumpets and rams' horns. They must have looked pathetic.

Has anyone ever teased you when you were trying to make a healthy choice with your eating, saying something like, "That's just rabbit food. Pretty soon you're gonna' start hopping around here." Have they laughed at you when you ordered your baked potato dry? Have they tried to bribe you off of your *Weigh to Win* Rainbow Food Plan by saying, "Just one little bite won't hurt you!" Were you embarrassed?

At first I was embarrassed to go into a restaurant and question everything on the menu. In 1986 there were not as many healthy choices to make in restaurants as there are now. If there was nothing baked or broiled on the menu, I would have to ask them to prepare something special for me. People do not believe this about me now, but underneath I have always been quite shy. It was embarrassing for me to make a special request, but I soon found restaurant employees to be very nice and cooperative with my requests. In fact, one restaurant where I liked to eat never listed anything on the menu as being baked or broiled, but they readily agreed to bake or broil any menu item for me any time I stopped in for a meal. Before long, the restaurant had new menus printed offering several choices of baked and broiled foods. I must not have been the only one "nervy" enough to make my wishes known.

☐ Fourth, the Israelites had to have perseverance. They had to march for seven days and nothing less would do. Do you think that if they had begged and pleaded, God would have relented and caused the wall to crumble in three days instead of seven? Maybe they could have bargained with God and compromised at five days? No, I do not think any amount of begging or bargaining would have changed the situation. God laid out the plan and nothing less would do.

We have to persevere with our weight loss journey, even if it takes years to accomplish the task. Begging God to remove our desire to eat, or pleading with Him to banish all the cookies from the face of the earth, will not get us to the end of our journey any sooner.

In the past, I would become impatient when I did not lose weight quickly. I wanted five to ten pounds off every week. Through my weight loss this time, I tried to be realistic. I tried not to think about how much weight I had to lose. I concentrated on making healthy food choices, instead. I was happy with any weight loss—even the quarter pound ones. As long as I was losing I was satisfied with my progress. Losing 120 pounds in a year sounds like a fast weight loss. Actually, it averages out to just a little over two pounds per week. When you are as large as I was, that kind of weight loss is gradual and realistic.

☐ Finally, the Israelites had faith that God was with them. They had faith even though they could not physically see the progress. Sometimes our weight loss is slow and we cannot see much progress, but we need to have faith that we are making progress, if we are doing our part.

I was so large that I had to lose thirty pounds before anyone even noticed, and then they were not really sure. The style of clothing I wore all had elastic in the waist so that I had to lose at least thirty pounds before any alterations were necessary. It took a lot of hard work to lose that first thirty pounds. I just had to have faith in myself and faith in God that I was doing the right thing. Progress was being made not only in my thinning body, but in the eating habits and learned behaviors which had kept me overweight so long.

Walls Test Our Faith

Sometimes walls are there to test our faith and teach us to be overcomers. We need to take steps to overcome.

☐ The first step is to be willing to take the step. Be available. Tell God, "I will be one of the people to march around that wall—I will do my part! Tell me what You want me to do—teach me, Lord." Or, you might say, "Lord, I am willing to do my part to change the lifestyle of overeating which has caused me to be overweight. I just ask You to be with me throughout the journey."

☐ The second step is to change your routine. Move out of the rut of indifference. Often God requires us to make a move before He steps in. Have you ever griped and complained as you gave up on yet another diet and said, "This is it. I am never going on a diet again"? I challenge you to move out of your rut of indifference. It really is a wall of protection which you build around you to keep the hurt of failure away. There is hope for you. By following the *Weigh to Win Weight Management System* you have made the first move. Continue to do your part and God will be there to help you. I believe in you too. You can succeed this time!

There Is Victory Ahead

The Israelites would have their victory—but only as they cooperated with God. We can be so hard to deal with and just plain stubborn. God knows what is best for us if we will let Him teach us. But He is not going to take problem foods out of our hands if we choose to eat them. It is not fair to stomp our feet and stubbornly say, "I want this chocolate chip cookie and I am going to eat it," and then blame God for not taking away our desire for chocolate chip cookies. If we show a spirit of cooperation by saying, "God, I am going to refuse the tray of chocolate chip cookies I see being passed around. Please help me to refuse," God will be there.

Joshua 6:20-21 proclaims, "When the trumpets sounded, the people shouted, and at the sound of the trumpet, when the people gave a loud shout, the wall collapsed; so every man charged straight in, and they took the city. They devoted the city to the Lord."

The best part is experiencing the victory. God never fails. Defeat is not in His plan. If you will do your part, He will not let you down!

I sure shouted the night that I reached my weight loss goal. I let out a whoop and cried with joy. I stood in front of my support group, shared the story of my wall of Jericho, and testified that March 16, 1987 was the day my wall came crashing down. I thanked God then, and I still thank Him for continuing to be there for me when I need Him, for continuing to teach me, for continually encouraging me. He is my closest Friend.

God wants us to be overcomers, if not presently, then ultimately. "In all these things we are more than conquerors through Him who loved us" (Romans 8:37). We are on the *winning* side.

> Success, success to you,
> and success to those who help you,
> for your God will help you.
> (1 Chronicles 12:18b)

What Weigh to Win Members Say

Since I consider weight loss to be a very private and personal accomplishment, you will not find the complete names or locations of the people who have willingly written these enthusiastic remarks about the *Weigh to Win Weight Management System*. As a Christian organization, we stand on our word that the following information is factual, with no one receiving compensation for their written support of our program.

May you find hope and encouragement from these words of success from others.

"I have finally accomplished my weight loss goal. I have tried for over thirty years to lose weight never to quite reach my goal. With the spiritual and emotional support from *Weigh to Win* and Lynn Hill, I have finally lost over seventy pounds. I know the continued support is there for me to maintain my weight loss. Thank God for *Weigh to Win.*"

—PEGGY *(lost 76 pounds)*

"To me *Weigh to Win* was a gift from God."
—JANET *(lost 113 pounds)*

"These prints are not very good, but I guess you can get an idea how much difference fifty pounds can make on a 5'1" body. I am thrilled with the difference it has made in my life. Thank you again for sharing this program with others. God bless you."

— BETH *(lost 50 pounds)*

"I look forward to using this plan to guide me in the way I eat for the rest of my life and also to use your encouraging, motivating, and inspirational material to help me keep living the way I am supposed to the rest of my life—depending on God's love instead of food to cope with struggles that everyone's life encounters. Thank you so much for making this program available."

— VIRGINIA *(lost 14 pounds)*

"I hope this will be of some help to you in return for the help that I have received from the *Weigh to Win* program. I have tried many diets and this is the first food plan that has fit my lifestyle and that I know, with God's help, I'll be able to incorporate into my daily living for the rest of my life whether I'm at home, at work, or on the road."

— ANONYMOUS

"*Weigh to Win* is an answer to my prayers. They have taught me to eat properly and to let God help me make wise choices because 'I can do everything through Him [Jesus Christ] who gives me strength (Philippians 4:13)."

— LORI *(lost 45 pounds)*

"I'm so thankful for *Weigh to Win*. . . . My reasons for 'taking the plunge' included doing it for myself, my health . . . and also I can be a better testimony for my

Lord. For the first time I'm losing weight without the 'crutch' of diet pills and it's great!"

—ANONYMOUS *(lost 25 pounds)*

"I'm enclosing our family picture. It's the first ever because I would never agree to have one made before I lost weight. I'm just so very thankful for you and the *Weigh to Win* program. Thank you."

—GLENDA *(lost 63 pounds)*

"A little bit at a time is how my weight is leaving me. Some weeks good, some weeks not so good, but hey, I didn't just all of a sudden have this overweight problem. It crept on a little at a time till my clothing size went up and up and up. Since joining *Weigh to Win,* I have learned many good, new eating habits and have thrown away many bad eating habits. Even tho' my weight is coming off very slowly, I'm eating healthier and feeling on top of the world. Doctors say crossing one's legs is bad for circulation, ha, I cross mine all the time because this is the first time in years one leg goes over the other so easily. When walking I hold my head up, shoulders back, chest out, thinking what a great world is all around me and how fortunate I am to be able to belong to this kind of program that helps to broaden my outlook on life, not my body. Do yourself a favor—try *Weigh to Win.*"

—SHIRLEY *(on her way)*

Medical Endorsements

"*Weigh to Win* does have at its foundation a very healthy and nutritionally complete exchange diet. This would be a good diet for all human beings to adhere to whether having problems with their weight or not. The *Weigh to Win* program incorporates education and encouragement for those working to establish a healthy diet and decrease and maintain an ideal body weight."

—DAVID M. ROSENTRATER, M.D.
Bremen, Indiana

"Since the '60s our American society has gone from 'thin is in' to 'fat is where it's at.' It is my opinion that if a person chooses a healthy, nutritionally balanced diet composed of the four basic food groups in moderate amounts daily that they will run less risk of health-related diseases. After extensively studying the *Weigh to Win* weight loss program, I am convinced that this program offers such a plan. It is my opinion that this program is a medically safe, sensible, and affordable approach to society's age-old problem of weight loss and control."

—PHILIP E. KELLAR, M.D.
Highland, Indiana

"Since I have carefully reviewed and continue to assess *Weigh to Win's* program, I know it a very safe plan for weight loss. I am really excited about *Weigh to Win's* approach. They are committed to sound nutritional practices and realistic weight loss goals."

—MARLA SMITH, R.D.
Member of the American Dietetic Assn.

Mission Statement

"*Weigh to Win* offers hope through education, compassion, and understanding. We are able to assist anyone seeking help with a weight management problem to learn a healthy eating lifestyle in an atmosphere of Christian love."

This mission statement is my commitment to you, dear friend. If you are ready to take that first step to a healthier body, I would like to help you.

Weigh to Win, Inc.
113 E. Washington
Suite 108
Plymouth, Indiana 46563
1-800-642-THIN

To purchase the complete *Weigh to Win Weight Management System* and supplemental resources, please visit your local Christian bookstore.

Endnotes

1. Eva May Nunnelley Hamilton, Eleanor Noss Whitney, and Frances Sienkiewicz Sizer, *Nutrition: Concepts and Controversies,* (St. Paul: West Publishing Company, 1988, 286-290). Adapted with permission.
2. Adapted with permission of Russell Pate, Ph.D., University of South Carolina, Columbia Human Performance Laboratory.
3. Hamilton, Whitney, and Sizer, *Nutrition: Concepts and Controversies,* 460-462.

For Further Reading

Cook, Shirley. *The Exodus Diet Plan,* Old Tappan, New Jersey: Fleming H. Revell Company, 1986.

Coyle, Neva, and Marie Chapian. *Free to Be Thin,* Minneapolis: Bethany House Publishers, 1979.

Coyle, Neva, and David Dixon. *Getting Your Family on Your Side,* Minneapolis: Bethany House Publishers, 1987.

Hamilton, Eva May Nunnelley, Eleanor Noss Whitney, and Frances Sienkiewicz Sizer. *Nutrition: Concepts and Controversies,* St. Paul: West Publishing Company, 1988.

McBarron, Janet, and J.T. Cooper. *The McBarron-Cooper Clinic-D Program,* Erie, Pennsylvania: Green Tree Press, Inc., 1987.

Minirth, Frank B., and Paul D. Meier. *Happiness Is a Choice,* Grand Rapids: Baker Book House, 1978.

Nash, Joyce D. *Maximize Your Body Potential: 16 Weeks to a*

Lifetime of Effective Weight Management, Palo Alto, California: Bull Publishing Company, 1986.

Satter, Ellyn. *How to Get Your Kid to Eat . . . But Not Too Much,* Palo Alto, California: Bull Publishing Company, 1987.

Stuart, Richard B. *Act Thin, Stay Thin,* New York: W.W. Norton and Company, 1978.

Thompson, Frank Charles. *The Thompson Chain-Reference Bible: New International Version,* Indianapolis: B.B. Kirkbride Bible Co., Inc.; Grand Rapids: Zondervan Bible Publishers, 1983.

Wise, Karen. *God Knows I Won't Be Fat Again!* Nashville: Thomas Nelson Inc., Publishers, 1978.